The Scientific Revolution in S

MW00364210

By Hannah Sivak, PhD

Cover illustration: *Madonna dell'Impannata (detail).* Raphael and Workshop. 1513-1514. Oil on wood. Palazzo Pitti, Florence.

Illustrations by Claire Thomas

Acknowledgements:

I wish to thank Andrea Still for her help with the manuscript.

I dedicate this book to my extraordinary family, for keeping me on my toes.

Thank you!

Hannah

Nature distributed medicine everywhere.

Gaius Plinius Secundus (Pliny the Elder) AD 23 - AD 79

Science is based on observation and experimentation as guided by the scientific method. Science is NOT guided by gut feelings, hunches, narratives or fancy stories.

Hannah Sivak, founder of Skin Actives Scientific

Thank you so much for your ongoing relationship with Skin Actives! Please enjoy this copy of Dr. Sivaks book, *The Scientific Revolution in Skin Care*, as a token of our appreciation.

Best wishes,
Dr. Hannah Sivak, Jonatan, & the Skin Actives Team

TABLE OF CONTENTS

Dear reader
Author's introduction: Hannah Sivak, PhD
The importance of healthy skin

- Sunlight is more than what we see
- Not everything UV light does to you is bad
- Oxidation and aging
- What is oxidative stress?
- ROS* initiate destructive chain reactions
- How bad is oxidative stress for your skin?
- Antioxidants: the scavengers of ROS*
- Plant sourced antioxidants
- Skin problems related to ROS*
- Non-enzymatic antioxidants
- How much oxygen do we want?
- What's so special about Skin Actives? The enzymatic scavengers of ROS*
- The most remarkable antioxidant product, unique to SAS: the ROS* Terminator
- Antioxidant Serum
- Antioxidant Day Cream
- Add individual antioxidants to your own formulation

- Myth: Sunblock/sunscreen completely protects your skin
- Skin pigmentation, a brief overview
- What does skin pigment do?
- Does dark skin require special care?
- Main causes of uneven pigmentation
- Aging
- Melasma
- Sun damage
- Post-inflammatory pigmentation
- Vitiligo
- Dark under eye circles
- How to avoid uneven pigmentation
- What to do after the fact
- What not to do
- SAS Skin Brightening Cream addresses multiple factors
- Pigmentation modifiers to avoid

Appendices (on Skin Actives Scientific website: skinactives.com)
- Ingredient Glossary (under the Resources tab)
- Our Science (on website footer)
- Dr. Sivak's Publications (in our Forum, under the Community tab)

Dear reader,

I assume that most of you will be reading this book jumping from what interests you to another bit that also interests you, and skipping the boring stuff. This is OK by me, but this is the reason why you will find repetitions here and there (and also there). This is because there are some issues that in my opinion are too important to let you leave this book without learning about. One example is the need for preservatives in skin care products, so don't be surprised if you see the same ideas in several sections.

Author's introduction: Hannah Sivak, PhD

My undergraduate studies were in Biology, specifically Plant Physiology. I did my doctorate research at the Institute for Biochemical Research in Buenos Aires, directed by Dr. L. F. Leloir, Nobel Laureate for Chemistry, 1970. My publications include one book on starch biochemistry and molecular biology, and more than 60 papers in international, refereed journals and in books, dealing with different aspects of biology, biochemistry, microbiology, molecular biology and biotechnology. I was a research fellow at the Universities of York and Sheffield, United Kingdom (1980-1990) and a Professor (Research) of Biochemistry and Molecular Biology at Michigan State University (1990-2002).

I was still a teenager when I entered university in Buenos Aires in 1966, and I fell in love with biology, which I had chosen as a major on a whim, like everything I did as a teen. I encountered a microscope when I was 18 and was excited to learn about plant anatomy, fungi, life cycles, photosynthesis and life in general. When I encountered the beauty of diatoms, minute algae with beautiful shapes, I decided to name any future daughter after diatoms (I didn't, and I'm sure my daughter is grateful for that). After years as a mediocre high school student, I became a top student in university; falling in love with science did that to me. The excitement of those years has never left me. I will never be bored with science; the joy of discovery and learning is what keeps me young.

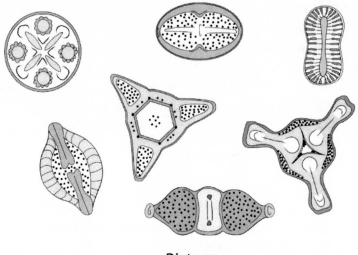

Diatoms

My life as a scientist started when I was a botany student, and to this day I follow the nomenclature rules instilled in me by Professor Arturo Burkart. Life at the biochemical laboratory actually started in 1976. Here's why: real life intruded on my love affair with science. I had a few very useful years as a plant physiologist, but was "purged" in December 1974, during a period of political repression by the government of Isabel Peron. After a hiatus of a couple of years, I was amazingly lucky to find refuge at the Research Institute directed by Nobel Prize winner Dr. Luis Leloir, and this changed my life forever. I'm so grateful to Dr. Leloir and my mentors, Dr. Carlos Cardini and Dr. Juana Tandecarz, for the opportunity they gave me to learn the craft at one of the best laboratories in the world, surrounded by good people. Biochemistry was a whole new world, where I could understand how nature works the way it does. I learned, at the molecular level, how plants make the chemicals that shape our world.

One of the most valuable tools I gained during my training at the Institute of Biochemistry Research (IIB) in Buenos Aires, was to learn how to read a scientific paper, i.e. how to isolate actual data from mere commentary and decide what conclusions could be drawn from the research. I also published my first papers in scientific journals. Scientific analysis is a tool I use when I choose actives to incorporate into our formulations on the basis of published scientific papers. I also use it to *translate* ingredient lists, separating what is actually in the formulation of expensive products from marketing gibberish. I also became familiar with everything related to polysaccharides such as beta glucans and more, you'll find them everywhere in our formulations.

In York and Sheffield, I gained expertise in the separation of plant subcellular organelles (you'll find cauliflower mitochondria in our Revitalizing Night Cream) and had new insights into the interaction between subcellular organelles. My scientific tourist visits to Seville, Spain gave me training in microalgae and a love for orange flowers. That time inspired a number of products with microalgae and a few with neroli, the essential oil extracted from petals of orange flowers.

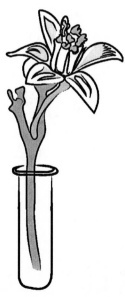

England was a welcome oasis to me, but scientists are a bit like soccer players: we move following professional opportunities. I had started moving back to "test tube biochemistry" and molecular biology in Sheffield, and now at Michigan State University, protein expression and characterization became my main interest. You will find special proteins in many of our products, and we also provide them to MDs for special formulations and projects. Some of my colleagues at MSU are now consultants for Skin Actives Scientific.

A few years ago I retired from academia and joined the "real world", applying decades of scientific research to practical matters. I had the opportunity to learn firsthand how the skin care industry works from the inside. In the industry, science is used mainly as a marketing tool, not as a practical guide for formulations. My son, with a background in physics and logistics, pushed me to start a business and do things my own way by putting science first. That is how Skin Actives got started.

When people ask me how I learned to do what I do, I have to say that it all started by watching my mother work in her kitchen - that, plus a passion for science, more than 40 years of learning from the best how to *do* science, long hours on the bench, and a willingness to listen to those who know more than I do.

This book will help you understand how your skin functions and changes. It will help you comprehend skin care ingredient lists; and what each ingredient does or does not do for you. I don't want anyone to be a sitting duck for the marketing departments that sell false promises in fancy packaging. Why not take your skin care into your own hands? You'll know exactly what you're doing.

The importance of healthy skin

For many people, their face and the *age their face projects* to the world, will determine whether they get a particular job or whether they get to the second date. We may not like it, but it's a fact. How we look is important. Even for those of us who don't go out much, our skin is incredibly important. If your life is good and you want to keep living it into your 90's, healthy skin will make an enormous difference. The paper-thin skin of the very old cannot do its job properly - keeping infectious agents out, keeping water in, etc., and it feels uncomfortable. There's no reason why aging should thin our skin to that extent; we should keep our skin not just *looking young*, but "working young". So often, a consumer will choose to undergo plastic surgery (where a doctor will stretch the skin, cut pieces of it away and insert fillers) or endure prescription injections to immobilize underlying muscles, without first thinking that the procedure as a whole might fail if the skin isn't really *healthy*.

From my experience in the skin care industry, I know how an *anti-aging* cream is planned, designed, manufactured, packaged, and sold. From my scientific experience I know what it will actually *do* when applied to the skin. Consumers of every background suspend their disbelief when it comes to skin care products. This is ridiculous. I want to provide you with a scientific understanding of skin care so you will know what's possible, what's not, and when to ignore the marketing altogether.

Chapter 1: Labels and ingredient lists

How to look at an ingredient list. First: don't panic!

The ingredient lists on the labels of skin care products look, at first sight, practically undecipherable, and probably just the same at second sight. And yet, it *is* possible to understand what's in that product if you really dive in. It helps if you know some chemistry, but if not, you can still work it out with patience, and if all else fails - you can write to me (SAS has a forum).

A good start is to try and separate the ingredients into two lists: a list of ingredients that make the *carrier*, be it a cream or serum, and a list of the *actives* dissolved in the cream or serum. For a very basic cold cream, you will find just a few components: water, mineral oil (very emollient, a skin *conditioner*), wax (a thickener), and fragrance. For a commercial product, the lists get longer because formulators use a variety of ingredients to improve *feel,* texture, stability and color.

For example, here is the list of ingredients for Skin Actives' Canvas Cream, a base cream that works well in many jobs. This formulation doesn't contain mineral oil, making it lighter and suitable for people with acne. We call it a base cream because we can modify it for any purpose (anti-acne, rejuvenating, etc.) by adding active ingredients. Each ingredient is followed by its purpose.

Note: Ingredients are presented here in lower case, and Latin names of the plants were removed to facilitate reading. INCI nomenclature capitalizes terms in the labels even when in scientific use this is not needed. When the binomial system (Linnaeus) is used, botanical rules are followed.

- water (formulation base)
- jojoba seed oil (emollient)
- sorbitol (water binding and slip, ease of application)

- butylene glycol (slip)
- cetyl alcohol (moisturizer and thickener)
- glyceryl stearate (moisturizer and thickener)
- PEG-100 stearate (moisturizer and thickener)
- stearyl alcohol (moisturizer and thickener)
- sesame seed oil (moisturizer)
- sweet almond oil (moisturizer)
- avocado oil (moisturizer)
- sodium hyaluronate (water binding, nutrient)
- polysorbate 20 (emulsifier)
- citric acid (to adjust pH)
- dimethicone (skin conditioner, slip agent)
- carbomer (thickener)
- aminoethyl propanol (antimicrobial preservative)
- phenoxyethanol (antimicrobial preservative)
- methylparaben (antimicrobial preservative)
- propylparaben (antimicrobial preservative)

If we look at a *cosmeceutical*, a skin care product formulated to rejuvenate the skin, things get even more complicated. Here we have the ingredients of the base cream and the actives mixed in the list and we have to go one by one to see what they are and what they are doing in the formulation. Also, the names come separated by just a comma, to save space on the label.

Water, glycerin, tetrahexyldecyl ascorbate, phosphatidylcholine, isopropyl palmitate, L-tyrosine, butylene glycol, glyceryl stearate, PEG-100 stearate, cetearyl alcohol, oligopeptide-17, ceteareth-20, magnesium aspartate, zinc gluconate, dimethylaminoethanol (DMAE), docosahexaenoic acid, ascorbyl palmitate, phenoxyethanol, dimethicone, caprylyl glycol, glycolic acid, retinyl palmitate, yeast ferment, palm oil, carbomer, disodium EDTA, tocotrienols, copper gluconate, polysorbate 20, sorbic acid, tocopherol, sodium hyaluronate, acetyl hexapeptide-8, palmitoyl oligopeptide, astaxanthin, palmitoyl tetrapeptide-3.

Why is this more complicated than the ingredient list for a cold cream (water, mineral oil, wax and fragrance)? There are several reasons, let's examine them.

The ingredients in the base cream have been changed into a more long-lasting, lighter formulation: water, glycerin, isopropyl palmitate, butylene glycol, glyceryl stearate, PEG-100 stearate, cetearyl alcohol, phenoxyethanol, dimethicone, caprylyl glycol, palm oil, carbomer, disodium EDTA, polysorbate 20, sorbic acid.

The list still includes oil and water, plus emulsifiers and thickeners. It also includes preservatives to extend the shelf life of the product: phenoxyethanol, disodium EDTA, polysorbate 20, sorbic acid. Mineral oil has been replaced by palm oil, glyceryl stearate, isopropyl palmitate, cetearyl alcohol, caprylyl glycol and dimethicone (a silicone), which will result in a lighter, less occlusive cream.

In this list there are chemicals that did not exist in the year 1900, they were created by chemists. Carbomer, a thickener, is an example; another is polysorbate 20, an emulsifier. Butylene glycol will help dissolve other ingredients. Many ingredients do double or triple jobs, but we can still identify them as solvents, thickeners, emulsifiers, and/or antimicrobial preservatives. You can find the chemical structure and function of each ingredient on the internet. Many university websites have their own educational sites, and Wikipedia is an excellent source for chemistry information. For example, Wikipedia gives this description of cetearyl alcohol: "cetostearyl alcohol, cetearyl alcohol or cetylstearyl alcohol is a mixture of fatty alcohols, consisting predominantly of cetyl and stearyl alcohols, and is classified as a fatty alcohol. It is used as an emulsion stabilizer, opacifying agent, and foam-boosting surfactant, as well as an aqueous and nonaqueous viscosity-increasing agent. It imparts an emollient feel to the skin and can be used in water-in-oil emulsions, oil-in-water emulsions, and anhydrous formulations.

It is commonly used in hair conditioners and other hair products."

Don't get discouraged by the technical description and the unknown names. Try to get a general idea of what the ingredient is and why it is present in the formulation. It would be nice to find all of these terms in a glossary on the internet, and you can, but often, instead of an actual definition, you will find advertising or a political agenda. Generic websites may be related to pressure groups that will try to convince you that many materials are *dangerous* based on their own vested interests and very non-scientific methods. Avoid them unless you know enough chemistry to tell what is information and what is misinformation.

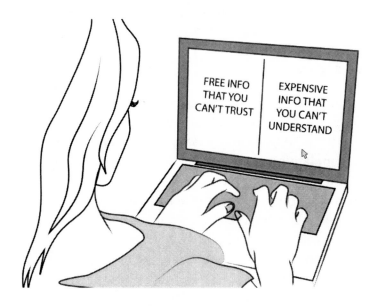

The perfect place to find all this information would be the INCI dictionary. Unfortunately, this dictionary, in several editions and now on-line, has been priced for the cosmetic industry by the organization that produces it, the Personal Care Products Council (PCPC, previously known as CTFA) at $1000 to $9000 per annual subscription. This is unfortunate, because the websites that are free and convenient for consumers to read are the ones offering scary definitions of ingredients (these websites belong to *non-profit* companies that make money by other means). The PCPC is adding information gradually on its new website, http://www.cosmeticsinfo.org. At the Skin Actives website (skinactives.com), we provide a glossary that includes the actives we use in our products, but the industry uses many thousands of ingredients and it's not practical to include them all.

So go ahead and use Wikipedia and with time you'll become familiar with most ingredient names, because most commercial products are variations of the same basic formulations. The novelty is generally reserved to the *actives*.

Formulation aids by function

 We at SAS are all about active ingredients, the components responsible for aiding the skin. But these actives require a good formulation, be it a liquid, lotion or cream, to do their job. To make a good formulation, many ingredients are mixed, according to their solubility and requirements, to achieve a homogeneous mix that will protect the actives and complement their action. Here are categories of ingredients that are used to create the carrier, or base of any product: solvents, butters and oils, emulsifiers, acidity adjusters, thickeners and preservatives.

A **solvent** is a liquid used to dissolve a powder; the solute dissolves because its molecules interact with the molecules of the solvent. Example: sugar will dissolve in water but not in oil. In skin care, solvents are ingredients that are used to dissolve other ingredients. They include water, vegetable or animal oils, silicones, alcohols, etc. When I plan a formulation, my objective is to use actives at the optimal concentration. If the active is not soluble in water or in oil, I may have to find an alternative solvent, because the skin will not absorb the un-dissolved active. In most SAS products, there are many actives so I may need a good mix of solvents (rather than just water) to give all those actives a chance to dissolve and stay dissolved.

The physical properties of an ingredient, including its capacity to dissolve in a particular solvent, are fixed. The capacity to dissolve depends on the relationships that the molecule can establish with the molecules of the solvent.

Finding the right solvent, or mix of solvents, is a craft. Tables in chemical indexes provide solubility information on a few solvents that are useful in the chemistry lab (water, ethanol, acetone), but of these only water is suitable for skin care use. It is up to the formulator to experiment until he/she gets a nice solution.

Floral waters are sometimes used instead of water; they are a byproduct in the production of essential oils by distillation. Floral waters are mostly water but some chemicals in the petals of the flowers used as source are also present in the floral water and they can give a very nice fragrance to the final product. "Floral water" also looks better on a label than plain old water.

Acidity adjusters are strong acids or bases added by the formulator to adjust the pH of the final product. During the preparation of the product, addition of various acids may decrease the pH too much, so towards the end the formulator will add some base, like sodium hydroxide or potassium hydroxide, to neutralize the acid and increase the pH of the product. The final pH should approximate the pH of the skin (near neutral pH, 7.0). Products with high (alkaline) or low pH (acidic) can damage the skin. Sometimes though, they can be useful, like in ascorbic acid serum.

Butters and oils are often present to add emolliency to products formulated for dry skin. The most common oils are those also used in foods (sunflower, maize, olive) but you will also see shea, tucuma, palmarosa oil, palm oil, pumpkin, wheat germ and many others. This is because the fatty acid composition varies between plant oils, making some more useful than others. Of course sometimes oils are chosen just because they look better on the ingredient list.

Emulsifiers. Water and oil don't mix, but an emulsifier can stabilize a suspension of two liquids that are not miscible. Emulsifiers are substances capable of relating to both water and fats, helping to make an emulsion, a dispersion of minute droplets of one liquid in the other.

Preservatives are ingredients that can kill or stop the growth of bacteria and mold present in the formulation or introduced during use of the product. Preservatives are usually mixes of chemicals because the mix has to stop different types of metabolisms of the organisms to be killed or stopped.

Thickeners are added to formulations to make them firmer, increase their viscosity and make the product more convenient or pleasant to use. We use a variety of thickeners that often have other functions in the formulations. Examples are xanthan gum, alginic acid and other polysaccharides and proteins.

Types of skin care products

Cream: an emulsion of oil and water in approximately equal proportions that penetrates well the outer layer of skin. Both oil soluble and water soluble actives can be used. Creams have a higher viscosity (thickness) than lotions.

Lotion: a low viscosity topical preparation.

Gel: a jelly-like material that can have properties ranging from soft and weak to hard and tough. By weight, gels are mostly liquid, yet they behave like solids because the polymers dissolved in the water form a three-dimensional cross-linked network within the liquid. It is the cross-linking within the fluid that gives a gel its structure and contributes to the adhesive stick. Because viscosity of the gel depends on the interaction between the solid and water, it can change greatly by adding even small amounts of salts or other ingredients.

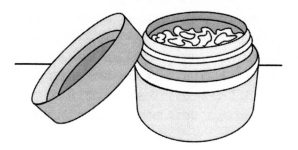

Our Sea Kelp Coral is an example of a gel

Serum: a (skin care industry) fancy term for lotion, with oil and water components that vary. Serum is a word borrowed from medicine, to suggest the idea of something strong that can benefit your skin. In medicine, the word refers to a blood-derived liquid, plasma, from which the clotting factors have been removed. The industry steals many terms from medicine and science in general. By FDA definition, a cosmetic cannot claim to change skin physiology. The medical-sounding terminology is used to convey the idea of medical benefits without annoying the FDA.

Sunscreen: a lotion that contains ingredients capable of absorbing or reflecting UV radiation before it reaches the skin thus preventing burning and photoaging. (Thankfully, the public has been educated about the dangers of sun exposure and tanning oil has all but disappeared from the market. The general population has evolved from wanting to promote or enhance a suntan to wanting to prevent tanning or burning. For skin that has seen too much sun and experienced sunburns, our UV Repair Cream will help.)

Toner is a liquid, mostly water but with additions, used to remove oils and sebum, stripping the skin of oily substances. Sebum, however, has a purpose: it lubricates skin and prevents water loss from the skin. People think that having oily skin means that the skin is dirty - this is not true at all. Photoshop has convinced people that the skin is supposed to be matte and not glossy.

Exfoliators remove dead skin cells to give skin a *smooth feel*. Be careful with exfoliation as there can be a cost to your skin. There are three ways of exfoliating your skin: physical *scrubs* (which involve a gritty texture that can come from sugar, salt, crushed nuts, crystals used in micro-exfoliation, etc.), chemical peels, and enzymatic peels. At Skin Actives we have products that use these three methodologies without resorting to brutal skin treatments that treat the skin as if it was an old wall in need of resurfacing by sandblasting. Welcome to the real world, where skin is not an inanimate object but a live organ, and knowledge is helpful; our constant goal at SAS is to preserve your skin's health.

Acid solutions, often called "chemical peels", break down the proteins in the most external layers of the skin when used with caution (if used without great caution they will burn the skin). Our TCA Spot Peel is the strongest we offer, for those clients' pesky hyperpigmentation spots that will not go away with anything else. Use as directed and you will do well. We have a milder form of chemical peel, our Alpha-Beta Exfoliator, which can be used on face, décolleté and hands without problems. It will provide an *invisible* peel, and you will have satisfyingly smooth skin without downtime or visible peeling. If you are looking for something even milder, our Vitamin C Serum with its low pH will leave your skin feeling smooth.

Labels 101

When choosing a recipe for a new dish to serve to my family, I consider many things, but by far the most important thing for me is the list of ingredients. A truly good product cannot be created out of bad ingredients. But with food, it *is* possible to create a *tasty* meal out of poor ingredients by loading up the dish with additives: sugars, fats, salt and monosodium glutamate (MSG), for example. Ingredients like those fool our brain into thinking we are eating something really great, when in reality it's not. The skin care industry works in a similar way, using advertising, fancy packaging and paid-for reviews as the equivalent of the fats and sugars in fast food. So how do we know whether a product is the skin care equivalent of a Big Mac or a Cordon Bleu dish? You can tell by reading the ingredient list. For both foods and cosmetics - it's really important to be able to read and understand ingredient labels!

Looking at a generic recipe for cold cream we can understand what's in it. Water, mineral oil, wax and fragrance. Things get complicated when we look at a commercial skin care product. When I look at the ingredient list of a skin care product, the list is an enumeration of the chemicals and plant extracts that make up the product, in order of concentration from the highest, usually water, to the lowest, often preservatives or fragrances and colorings. Let's take a look at the ingredient list for a product that is currently on the market (marketed as "Award-winning, patented technology powers this comprehensive anti-aging treatment, delivering dramatic, personal results for visibly smoother, firmer, radiant-looking skin.") for over $150 an ounce:
Water, glycerin, tetrahexyldecyl ascorbate, phosphatidylcholine, isopropyl palmitate, L-tyrosine, butylene glycol, glyceryl stearate, PEG-100 stearate, cetearyl alcohol, oligopeptide-17, ceteareth-20, magnesium aspartate, zinc gluconate, dimethylaminoethanol (DMAE), docosahexaenoic acid, ascorbyl palmitate, phenoxyethanol, dimethicone, caprylyl glycol, glycolic acid, retinyl palmitate, yeast ferment, palm oil, carbomer, disodium

EDTA, tocotrienols, copper gluconate, polysorbate 20, sorbic acid, tocopherol, sodium hyaluronate, acetyl hexapeptide-8, palmitoyl oligopeptide, astaxanthin, palmitoyl tetrapeptide-3.

This is the way I deal with the long and complicated ingredient lists. First I cross out the common components that make up the base (a stable emulsion, or blend, containing preservatives that will ensure that the actives are in a safe and stable carrier cream, serum or lotion). Water and glycerin are solvents (substances used for dissolving other substances) and will also provide hydration to your skin, a very useful property especially in winter and in air-conditioned environments. Isopropyl palmitate is a thickener and an emollient. Butylene glycol is another solvent, helping dissolve ingredients that water and glycerol cannot dissolve. There are more emulsifiers, solvents and thickeners than in cold cream. The reason for this complexity has to do with what the formulator is trying to achieve: a smooth mixture with a nice texture and feel that will keep the actives well dissolved and stable.

Here's the ingredient list with the components that make up the base crossed out:

~~Water~~, ~~glycerin~~, tetrahexyldecyl ascorbate, phosphatidylcholine, ~~isopropyl palmitate~~, L-tyrosine, ~~butylene glycol~~, ~~glyceryl stearate~~, ~~PEG-100 stearate~~, ~~cetearyl alcohol~~, oligopeptide-17, ~~ceteareth-20~~, magnesium aspartate, zinc gluconate, dimethylaminoethanol (DMAE), docosahexaenoic acid, ascorbylpalmitate, ~~phenoxyethanol~~, ~~dimethicone~~, ~~caprylyl glycol~~, glycolic acid, retinyl palmitate, yeast ferment, ~~palm oil~~, ~~carbomer~~, ~~disodium EDTA~~, tocotrienols, copper gluconate, ~~polysorbate 20~~, ~~sorbic acid~~, tocopherol, sodium hyaluronate, acetyl hexapeptide-8, palmitoyl oligopeptide, astaxanthin, palmitoyl tetrapeptide-3.

Next, the useful ingredients are **bolded**:

~~Water, glycerin~~, tetrahexyldecyl ascorbate,
phosphatidylcholine, ~~isopropyl palmitate~~, L-tyrosine,
~~butylene glycol~~, ~~glyceryl stearate~~, ~~PEG-100 stearate~~,
~~cetearyl alcohol~~, oligopeptide-17, ~~ceteareth-20~~, **magnesium**
aspartate, **zinc** gluconate, dimethylaminoethanol (DMAE),
docosahexaenoic acid, ascorbyl palmitate,
~~phenoxyethanol~~, ~~dimethicone~~, ~~caprylyl glycol~~, ~~glycolic
acid~~, **retinyl palmitate**, yeast ferment, ~~palm
oil~~, ~~carbomer~~, ~~disodium EDTA~~, **tocotrienols**, copper gluconate,
~~polysorbate 20~~, ~~sorbic acid~~, **tocopherol, sodium hyaluronate**,
acetyl hexapeptide- 8, palmitoyl oligopeptide, **astaxanthin**,
palmitoyl tetrapeptide-3.

Finally, I <u>underline</u> ingredients that can damage the skin in one
way or another (Another harmful ingredient very commonly
used in skin care is denatured alcohol).

~~Water, glycerin~~, tetrahexyldecyl ascorbate,
phosphatidylcholine, ~~isopropyl palmitate~~, L-tyrosine,
~~butylene glycol~~, ~~glyceryl stearate, PEG-100 stearate~~,
~~cetearyl alcohol~~, oligopeptide-17, ~~ceteareth-20~~, **magnesium**
aspartate, **zinc** gluconate, dimethylaminoethanol
(DMAE), **docosahexaenoic acid, ascorbyl palmitate,**
~~phenoxyethanol, dimethicone~~, ~~caprylyl glycol~~, ~~glycolic
acid~~, **retinyl palmitate**, yeast ferment, ~~palm oil~~, ~~carbomer~~,
~~disodium EDTA~~, **tocotrienols**, <u>copper gluconate</u>,
~~polysorbate 20~~, ~~sorbic acid~~, **tocopherol, sodium hyaluronate**,
acetyl hexapeptide- 8, palmitoyl oligopeptide, **astaxanthin**,
palmitoyl tetrapeptide-3.

What did we find out?
This product contains two vitamin C derivatives: tetrahexyldecyl
ascorbate and ascorbyl palmitate. For our SAS formulations I
prefer to use a stable water soluble vitamin C derivative like

magnesium ascorbyl phosphate. Tetrahexyldecyl ascorbate has not been proven to work as a vitamin C, but there seems to be evidence that ascorbyl palmitate does. Glycolic acid will do nothing for this product; to do its job it needs to be present at a high concentration and to be non-neutralized.

From the ingredients in the list, I like phosphatidyl choline, a useful lipid (fat) present in lecithin (and in Skin Actives' ELS - Every Lipid Serum). We also use DMAE, but with prudence because its mechanism of action is unknown. Docosahexaenoic acid, an unsaturated fatty acid, is the active in *Schizochytrium* oil (which is in ELS). Retinyl palmitate is vitamin A. We also use the antioxidants tocotrienol, tocopherol (the natural form—the synthetic mix can cause allergies), and astaxanthin. We use hyaluronic acid in all our creams and water-based serums. Why is the copper salt underlined? We avoid copper except in products used to aid healing, because excess copper can promote protein breakdown. As for synthetic peptides, very fashionable, we skip all those justified by the industry on the basis of weak research done in commercial laboratories. The sequences of most of those peptides are undisclosed, and I don't like *mystery ingredients*.

Careful reading of the ingredient list suggests that what we have here is a product that will work at firming the skin because it contains DMAE. It will also provide some nutrition (phosphatidyl choline, docosohexaenoic acid, L-tyrosine, etc.) and antioxidants. The retinoid also means that it will help somewhat to promote skin renewal. In short, this is not a bad product, and the packaging looks nice. But at over $150 for an ounce, is it really worth using?

My recommendation in this case: instead of trying to do so many things with one product, use our Vitamin A Cream at night, our Vitamin C Serum once or twice a week, and our DMAE Serum sparingly for special occasions. If you have dry skin, use ELS on its own; if not, you can add it to our Canvas Base Cream. These

products will provide much better results, and you'll have enough
money left over to go to a fancy restaurant!

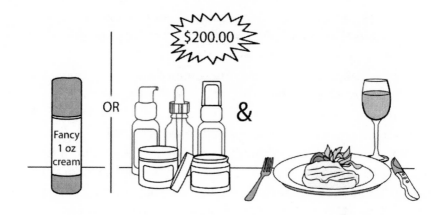

Silly ingredient lists

Sometimes ingredient lists aren't straightforward. Often, I have
to *translate* the list, as many ingredients are hidden behind a
Wizard of Oz curtain of scientific-sounding names. For translating,
I often use Google, a process that will highlight misspellings. An
ingredient being misspelled on a label can be unintentional, but on
occasion, misspelling is used to hide an unsavory ingredient. If the
ingredient is a plant extract, I may be familiar with the plant - I
was *raised* as a botanist; if not, I search the literature looking for
scientific research suggesting that the extract contains valuable
chemicals that may influence human skin physiology for
the *better* (many plant chemicals are actually poisonous).

Here are some examples: the sophisticated term *nikkomulese 41*
hides the less exciting mix of behenyl alcohol, polyglyceryl-10
pentastearate, and sodium stearoyl lactylate. *Fruit flower complex
12* is just that, a mystery complex. Who knows what's in it?
Simulgel is a mix of hydroxyethyl acrylate/ sodium
acryloyldimethyltaurate copolymer, isohexadecane, and

polysorbate 60. That product in the pretty jar that sells for hundreds of dollars sounds less attractive now, right?

Sometimes an ingredient is immune to searches entirely. When I tell readers that I can't comment on the possible benefits of alguronic acid - it's because alguronic acid doesn't exist. What does this mean? Alguronic acid does not appear in any scientific publication or Merck index. *Detective work* using the INCI (International Nomenclature for Cosmetic Ingredients) shows that the name does not lead to a defined chemical. If there is no definition of the term that leads to a clear composition, it's not possible to comment on it meaningfully. Commercial laboratories giving "independent" evaluations are not trustworthy as there is no peer review or methodology that allows scientists to try to duplicate the experiments and see whether the findings are correct. Apparently, alguronic acid has now been registered as a trade name, but using a scientific-sounding name shows that the intention was to confuse consumers.

Alguronic acid is a new addition to the *walk of shame* ingredients like *torricellumn*, *amatokin polypeptide #153*, *idebenol* and many others. These are ingredients that exist only in the imagination of marketers.

Usually, there is a concordance among the ingredients in the list. If one ingredient sounds like pseudoscience, "structured water", for example, the whole ingredient list is likely to be mostly junk.

Sometimes an ingredient looks interesting and I will read everything there is about it to see whether we should add it to our own products. Because many chemicals are present in a plant extract, I make sure that there are no reports of dangerous chemicals accompanying the "good" one. It's also important to choose the right part of the plant. For example, coleus essential oil is extracted from the leaves of the coleus plant and has antibacterial properties (specifically anti-acne), while forskolin is extracted from the root.

Though they come from the same plant, the chemical components are totally different and so is the activity. You will find these and many more ingredients described in our Ingredients Glossary, which is under the resources tab on the homepage (www.skinactives.com/Glossary.html).

Color and scent

There's a good reason why Skin Actives products don't look the same as most of the products sold in department stores. Some of the extracts we use have strong pigments or scents. A product ingredient list may contain fifty great ingredients, but if it's white in color or doesn't have a natural scent (or if every product made by a brand smell completely the same), you can assume that the *concentration of the useful ingredients is very low*. This is especially true of products billed as "natural" or "organic". The rules guiding ingredient lists allow this because the ingredients are listed in order of concentration until they reach one percent. Ingredients making up one percent or less of the product can be listed in any order.

"Label value"

The *less-than-1%* rule opens the door to "label value" ingredients, i.e. ingredients added at such low concentrations that they cannot exert any effect (good or bad) on the skin. But they look impressive on the label! This strategy is used for marketing purposes with ingredients that are extraordinarily expensive, have strong smells or colors that would affect the appearance of the product, or are insoluble in solvents compatible with skin physiology.

Once the ingredient list has been decoded and simplified, we can finally make an educated decision as to whether the product can do what the marketing materials say it can.

Limitations of the INCI nomenclature

The International Nomenclature of Cosmetic Ingredients, abbreviated INCI, is a system of names for ingredients of soaps and cosmetics. INCI names are mandated on the ingredient statement of every consumer personal care product, allowing the consumer to identify the ingredient content. The nomenclature is very useful.

For pure chemicals, the nomenclature is loosely based on scientific names. In the case of botanical extracts it relies on the botanical names (genus and species) of the plants, following the typical binomial Linnaean nomenclature, accompanied by the common name.

In some instances, INCI names may differ greatly from the systematic chemical nomenclature or from more common trivial names. Recently, I had my first direct contact with the INCI system, and I thought our clients would be interested to hear about how the system works. For a long time I have been complaining about the nomenclature for proteins, because it doesn't relate to the scientific nomenclature. I blamed the companies requesting an INCI name for a new ingredient. Well, I was wrong. I requested the very meaningful name "glutaredoxin" for the protein that scientists call "glutaredoxin". The name assigned by the Personal Care Products Council? Sh-Polypeptide-77. For our own products, we've decided to use the name glutaredoxin, because ingredient lists are supposed to inform the users, not confuse them.

A preservative by any other name (or no name) ...

"What's in a name? That which we call a rose
By any other name would smell as sweet."
    Romeo and Juliet (II, ii, 1-2)

True for roses, but what applies to roses does not necessarily apply to skin care. A prospective client wrote to me demanding to know why we at Skin Actives Scientific continue to use preservatives in our products when she has been doing so well with products that contain no preservatives whatsoever. My answer: the products you've been buying *do* contain preservatives. Why doesn't the consumer know this? In a battle that involves pressure groups, environmental politics, fear and marketing, the first casualty is science. The existence of the FDA rules and the INCI nomenclature may suggest that everything used in manufacturing the product must be listed on the label, but this is not always true.

Ways to hide preservatives from the consumer

Hide them in plain sight. The preservatives in the formulation are presented as emollients, or skin tighteners, or essential oils, or anything else but what they are: preservatives. This is possible for ingredients that aren't familiar to the consumer.

Confuse the consumer. The preservatives are not explicitly included in the list, but are included (and unmentioned) in the "natural" extracts. For example, if licorice root is extracted with a solution made of water, propylene glycol and preservatives such as parabens, all that needs to appear in the ingredient list for the final product is *licorice extract*. Moreover, if the plant was grown without synthetic fertilizers, herbicides or pesticides, the extract (which is mostly water, propylene glycol, and preservatives) can appear on the label as *organic licorice extract*. If plant extracts are a large part of the final product, no further preservatives will be needed, because the concentration of preservatives contributed by the *extracts* to the final product will be enough for safe preservation.

Lie. A company adds preservatives and simply lies about the formula. Yes, it happens. Unless somebody sends the product to an analytical laboratory to be tested, at a cost of several hundred dollars, nobody will be any wiser.

Let's look at the ingredient list of a product sold as a "preservative-free" "Restorative Night Moisture Cream":

water, glycerin, dimethicone, butylene glycol, diglycerin, C12-15 alkyl lactate, hydrogenated soybean oil, pentylene glycol, rose flower water, isopropyl palmitate, glyceral stearate, steareth-21, rice bran oil, squalane, steareth-2, caprylic/capric/myristic/stearic triglyceride, polysorbate 20, stearic acid, polysilicone-11, polysorbate 60, hydroxyethyl acrylate/sodium acryloyldimethyl taurate copolymer, white mulberry bark extract, aloe leaf juice, mallow flower extract, jojoba leaf extract, Japanese big leaf magnolia bark extract, fireweed flower/leaf/stem extract, honeysuckle flower extract, palmitoyl oligopeptide, palmitoyl tetrapeptide-7, carbomer, bentonite, xanthan gum, alanyl glutamine.

There are no obvious preservatives listed, but that doesn't mean they're not there. A mix of water, glycerin and other ingredients would start the process of decomposition soon enough, and shelf life (time available to sell a product before the smell and color changes considerably) would be measured in weeks, not the year required for the type of distribution system most brands need. The manufacturers say that their product is preservative-free, but preservatives are there, hidden as "process aids" which they don't have to declare on the label. The product is *not* free of preservatives, only the label is.

I wouldn't buy any product that claims to be "preservative-free" unless it's oil-based or because its composition (like the extreme pH in our trichloroacetic solution) precludes microbial growth. Otherwise, you are either buying a dishonest product or a dangerous one.

Please note that many essential oils have some antimicrobial activity; we use some of them in our acne control products. This doesn't mean that essential oils can carry the responsibility of preserving a nutrient-rich skin care product; at the concentrations required for preservation, the formula would be too irritating to the skin.

In short, preservatives, i.e. chemicals added to the formula for the purpose of killing or delaying growth of bacteria and mold, are always present in any formula, whatever the label may say. The notable exception is products completely free of water, because microorganisms need water to grow and divide. Skin Actives' Alpha Beta Exfoliator, Cleansing Oil, and Every Lipid Serum are formulated without water and therefore need no preservatives.

Chapter 2: The scientific revolution in skin care: from cold cream to cosmeceuticals

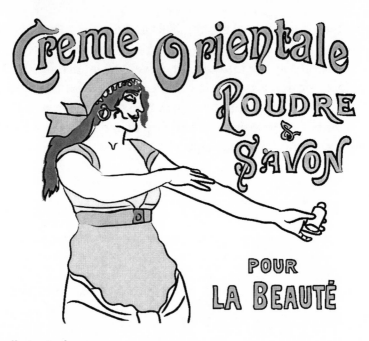

How it all started

"Take of white wax four ounces, oyl of roses omphacine a pound; melt in a double vessel, then powr it out into another, by degrees putting in cold water, and often powring it out of one vessel into another, stirring it till it be white; last of all wash it in rose water, adding a little rose water and rose vineger."

—*Nicholas Culpeper (b. 1650), London Dispensatory,* recounted in Moore, J. B. (1869). "On Cold Cream." American Journal of Pharmacy.

It is easy to see that something has changed in the world of skin care: in the beauty section of the fancy stores the jars are still beautiful and the creams inside smell so nice. But the advertising has changed; they discuss enzymes, peptides, glycans, telomerase and stem cells. The scientific revolution in skin care is here, but what does it all mean?

Once upon a time, there was cold cream. Cold cream is an emulsion of water, oils and beeswax used to smooth and protect the skin. The invention of cold cream is believed to be thousands of years old. How did we get from cold cream to the thousands of skin care products that inundate the supermarket, the pharmacy, and department stores? Although the advertising uses scientific verbiage, it is important to know that it was not the scientists who brought scientific discoveries to the industry, but the industry itself. What they did was add to the cream chemicals capable of changing skin physiology, giving cold cream (up to then a cosmetic) the capacity of not just improving the look of the skin but also to rejuvenate it. In theory, what the industry does is not allowed by the FDA.

Defining the word - cosmetic

There are many different definitions of what a cosmetic is or isn't, but the definition that holds the most importance for our industry comes from the Federal Drug and Cosmetic Act. As per Sec. 201(i) FD&C Act: "A cosmetic is a product, except soap, intended to be applied to the human body for cleansing, beautifying, promoting attractiveness or altering the appearance." The FD&C Act defines cosmetics by their intended use, as "articles intended to be rubbed, poured, sprinkled, or sprayed on, introduced into, or otherwise applied to the human body." Among the products included in this definition are: "skin moisturizers, perfumes, lipsticks, fingernail polishes, eye and facial makeup, cleansing shampoos, permanent waves, hair colors, and deodorants, as well as any substance intended for use as a component of a cosmetic product." According to Senate Report No. 493 and court decisions, the term *intended* in the legal definition of the term cosmetic means: "with respect to the use of a product, its directed or prescribed use as determined from the statements made on a product's label or labeling."

A cosmetic "is also a drug when it is intended to cleanse, beautify or promote attractiveness as well as treat or prevent disease or otherwise affect the structure or any function of the human body"

(Sec. 201(g) and (i), FD&C Act; Sec. 509, FD&C Act). The FD&C Act defines drugs as "products that cure, treat, mitigate or prevent disease". The key is the difference between altering the appearance (*cosmetic*) vs. affecting a disease (*drug*). Why is this distinction so important for manufacturers? While cosmetics don't require FDA approval prior to sale, drugs are subject to a costly and lengthy review and approval process by FDA.

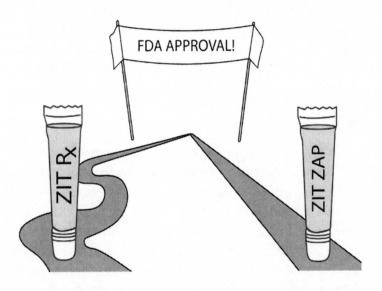

For a company to submit a new chemical to the FDA as a candidate for a drug designation there must be good reason to believe that the chemical will make money for the company. The chemical should be patentable and have a good possible market. If these conditions are not met, or if the company can't show data proving there are medical benefits, there's no point going through the expensive FDA authorization procedure.

What is a cosmeceutical?

Following the FDA's definition, a cosmetic is not supposed to have a physiological effect on the skin, yet millions of dollars are spent every day selling us products *because* they have a physiological effect on our skin: erasing wrinkles, increasing elasticity, lightening the skin, etc. But if a product has drug properties, it must be approved as a drug. What is going on here? The industry decided to navigate this very narrow gap by inventing a new term, *cosmeceutical*. While the FD&C Act does not officially recognize the term "cosmeceutical," the cosmetic industry uses this word to refer to cosmetic products that have medicinal or drug-like benefits, which by definition would make them drugs and subject to approval by the FDA.

The FDA allows for this imaginary gap as long as the public's health is not damaged and as long as claims on the labels or advertising don't try to dupe potential buyers into thinking that they're getting a medicine that is *proven* to do what it advertises. A new word was invented to cover ingredients and products that may have beneficial effects on the skin but whose manufacturers prefer not to call them drugs (medications). Why? The rules covering medications are onerous in many different ways. They must be manufactured in specially designed facilities, the formulations are carefully regulated and the claims must be proven in a way that satisfies the FDA requirements.

This is a gray area *by choice*. It allows skin care companies to innovate and allows the FDA to pretend that it is not happening. The result is that many cosmeceuticals are as effective as products sold as medications. The unspoken agreement is that products sold as cosmetics involve no danger to the consumer so there is no need of supervision by an MD.

The transition from cold cream to cosmeceuticals did not happen in a void. There have also been changes in the dietary supplement industry. In the USA Congress deregulated the businesses with the

Dietary Supplement Health and Education Act of 1994, allowing for the unlimited growth of a multibillion dollar industry that clearly affects the biochemistry and physiology of the whole body. Dietary supplements have easily jumped into cosmetics and just as some chemicals used in dietary supplements are useful, so they are when applied topically in creams or "serums". Expect changes in the future, as the FDA tries to catch up with the industry.

Because the system is not perfect (nor was it designed to be) loopholes are huge and allow bad products to get through. When they are caught, there is a big brouhaha but in the meantime the company playing the system laughs all the way to the bank. A big "no-no" is the use of prescription drugs in the formulation of products sold as cosmetics, and the most flagrant violation of this rule is the use of prostaglandin analogs (present in a prescription drug used to treat glaucoma) in eyelash "cosmetics". Although a big company was fined for this glaring infraction, others followed.

The products that don't break the law and fit within this gap could be defined as containing ingredients that are known to modify skin physiology but are not listed by the FDA as prescription or non-prescription medications. For example, products containing chemicals listed by the FDA as benefiting acne-affected skin cannot be sold as cosmetics. And yet, there's another loophole: you may be able to sell these products as cosmetics as long as the products do not *claim* to be "anti-acne".

The International Nomenclature of Cosmetic Ingredients lists ingredients that have a physiological effect as *skin modifiers*. Is this a serious limitation? Not really. It works as an encouragement to find better options than what is already on the market. This is the case with chemicals sold as medication for the skin but that have negative side effects that make them double-edged swords, like hydroquinone, benzoyl peroxide and topical antibiotics. Here you see a basic contradiction between the government and the skin care industry. There is no loophole but by using great care in advertising and labels the industry gets away with selling products that affect the function of the skin (part of the human body) while avoiding presenting them as drugs. Why is this useful? For the manufacturer, it saves money, because the cost, in time and money, of getting a prescription drug to the market is very high, and most chemicals are not patentable. For the consumer, this can result in a product that is effective, has no side effects and is less expensive than a prescription medicine.

I'm sure that people at the FDA are fully aware of this contradiction, as shown by the cases that come up in FDA inspections and legal action. One such action was that against the fraudulent "eyelash growth factor", a non-existing name that was hiding an actual medication (drug) used to control glaucoma. This is a clear example of misbranding and the FDA has produced reports and has put that company on notice.

The FDA also acts when a "cosmetic" harms a consumer. The manufacturer of the cosmetic product is responsible for ensuring that the product is safe.

What is Skin Actives Scientific? What do we mean by "active"?

SAS works in the narrow band between cosmetics and drugs. We don't use any chemicals listed as "Prohibited & Restricted Ingredients" by the FDA.

Without using a new word, we use the rather generic term *active* defined as a chemical, natural or synthetic, that can promote skin health and improve skin appearance and is *not* classified as a drug by the FDA.

Thinking about plastic surgery? Try some actives first

Thinking of getting plastic surgery? Or a laser procedure, or a drastic chemical peel? Stop and think Skin Actives first. You may think that drastic intervention is the way to make a big difference to your skin, but with drastic intervention comes a high risk of *messing up* your skin. There are alternatives! Before you take that path, make sure you first try the route that involves coaching your skin into making positive changes with the help of the actives that we provide.

One example - after a couple of months using our Vitamin A Cream and Collagen Serum, you may not need blepharoplasty (eyelid surgery). Not only is the cost of the surgery extremely high ($5,000 or more), so is the risk of the intrusion, cutting, and removing tissue.

Chapter 3: Myths and legends in the skin care industry

The skin care industry is full of myths and legends. Publicists are always looking for the story that will sell a new but otherwise unremarkable product as *special*. Maybe you're familiar with the story of the NASA scientist who discovered that fermented sea kelp could heal his awful scars, or the story about the soft and youthful hands of aged sake brewers. But these myths and legends are common to advertising and shouldn't be taken seriously. It is no different from using a pretty jar or a fancy French name on a label. They are silly but they can't hurt you. Some myths, however, are not that innocent.

Myth: Our skin is impermeable

If the skin were impermeable, you clearly would need the *delivery system* consisting of those nanoparticles designed by that famous scientist in Switzerland. Unfortunately, that famous scientist in Switzerland doesn't exist, or never published anything in a reputable scientific journal. More importantly, he is lying about skin properties: the skin is not impermeable and you don't need any delivery system to get an active into your skin. Whatever you apply to the skin will be absorbed, for better and/or worse. The outermost layer of the skin, the stratum corneum, limits water loss from the body to the environment and allows us humans, organisms that depend totally on water, to walk around in the Arizona desert and still be able to live. The stratum corneum also limits penetration of water and chemicals *into* the skin, slowing absorption of nutrients (and noxious chemicals) applied topically. "Limits penetration" doesn't mean that this layer is impermeable, as shown by water loss through the epidermis (trans-epidermal water loss or TEWL). Water loss across the skin can be measured easily with a laboratory instrument, and it increases with age and skin damage. In skin aged by sun exposure, absorption of external nutrients will be higher than in young skin, just like trans-epidermal water loss is higher.

The absorption of water-soluble nutrients through the skin will increase with skin humidity, so it's a good idea to take advantage of the skin's higher permeability after a shower or bath. Amino acids are electrically charged molecules, but when delivered in a cream, an emulsion of water and oil containing other nutrients and salts, this property should not preclude penetration. This reasoning led to our using the amino booster in an easily-applied cream rather than a serum. Even a low uptake of amino acids applied topically should substantially improve the health of skin deprived of nutrients by the decrease of blood supply to the dermis that occurs to all of us when we age. And this is valid for all useful actives applied topically: you don't need to absorb 100% of them, so forget about *delivery systems*. You don't need them, your skin is permeable enough.

Myth: Preservatives are bad for you

"How come other companies can make preservative-free products and Skin Actives can't?" We hear this question a lot, mostly from potential clients for private label products. We are asked to formulate skin care products that are effective, natural, organic, and free of preservatives. There are a multitude of companies selling skin care products advertised as pure, green, natural, and free of synthetic substances. There is complementary advertising posing as information, informing the public that the world is full of synthetic poisons and that it is time to go back to the gentle past when we relied on Mother Nature to take care of us. When I'm asked "how do they do it?"- I explain that they don't, the advertising just lies.

Is "preservative free" possible? Yes. You can use olive oil on your skin and it will provide fatty acids that skin can use. There's no need for preservatives, but be aware that pure olive oil does go rancid, via oxidization, after a few months. Note: if you have a bottle of extra virgin olive oil (E.V.O.O.) that is older than a year and it hasn't gone rancid, then it isn't what it says it is!

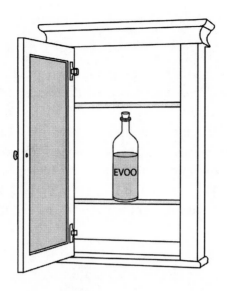

Conversely, any product containing water needs preservatives to prevent growth of bacteria and mold. It's not possible to sell skin care products containing water and nutrients without using preservatives. Skin Actives' Cleansing Oil and Alpha-Beta Exfoliator are preservative-free because they don't contain water, so they don't need preservatives. Most of the extracts we use at Skin Actives are powder extracts, dry and free of water, so there's no need to add preservatives until the extracts are mixed into a cream or a water-based serum. If you mix water and hyaluronic acid and forget to add a preservative, in a few days you'll see how the gel becomes a liquid as bacteria and mold consume the hyaluronic acid, breaking down the molecule and using it as food.

At Skin Actives we are very open about our preference for parabens as safe and effective preservatives at low concentrations. We also provide our European Cream which contains a different preservative called Optiphen Plus (phenoxyethanol, caprylyl glycol and sorbic acid). We list all of our ingredients on our website and we ensure that the ingredients in each product are used at effective concentrations. They're not there to look good on the label; they're there to help your skin.

Myth: Your skin care products should be organic

The word *organic* conveys a meaning of wholesomeness. When used for food, it means that the crop has been grown without adding synthetic fertilizers and no pesticides have been used. The FDA has some rules about how to use the word for food products, but when it comes to cosmetics, there are no rules. Many irresponsible companies will take advantage of the consumer, because no rules means no punishment. My advice: whenever you see the word "organic" in a skin or hair care product, look at the ingredient list and make sure you know how to read it.

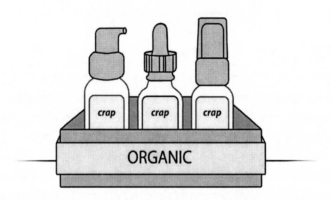

Here is the ingredient list for an anti-aging moisturizer from a brand whose name contains the word "Organics" – it is their "Coconut Age Corrective Moisturizer": coconut water, corn oil, cetearyl glucoside, cetearyl alcohol, shea butter, glycerin, chicory root oligosaccharides, tara tree gum, gluconolactone, grape seed oil, caprylic/capric triglyceride, stearic acid, coconut oil, carrot extract, squalane, coenzyme Q10, tocopheryl acetate, ascorbyl palmitate, apple fruit cell culture extract, lecithin, benzyl alcohol, xanthan gum, methyl glucose sesquistearate, salicylic acid, sodium benzoate, potassium sorbate, coconut fragrance.

The oils in this list may be certified organic because such certification exists, but I would say that the "Organics" in the name is there to obfuscate the facts and make the consumer forget that this is a mediocre formulation (and with a predominance of synthetic ingredients). Coconut water contains useful nutrients, but corn oil lacks the essential fatty acids your skin needs. Benzoic acid, sodium benzoate, and potassium sorbate are preservatives, and more are likely present in the coconut water, carrot extract, and "apple fruit cell culture extract". So the word *Organics* in their name garners your purchase and your trust - when the product is sub-par altogether. Buy organic cosmetics if you like to throw away extra money. Or you can find a company that makes well designed (using actives at the proper concentration) products that are supported by science, so you know the products will be effective.

Myth: Natural is good, synthetic is bad

Just two words: *stinging* nettle. Two more words? *Poison* oak. Plants can't run, and they have too many predators, starting with humans. To defend themselves they produce chemicals that will stop animals from eating them. *Natural* has become a buzzword, often empty of any meaning. For example: "allantoin from comfrey" in an ingredient list. Though it is true that you can find allantoin in comfrey, the ingredient used in skin care products is more likely to be synthetic. Not that it matters - the chemical extracted from the plant cannot be distinguished from the synthetic one, but this approach only perpetuates this myth that natural is better than synthetic.

What is natural? It can be defined as a substance found in nature that hasn't been chemically transformed. Purification that involves simple physical procedures is allowed; it does not change the original chemical. Here, I would like to present you with a dishwashing liquid I saw on the kitchen counter of a family member. It looks lovely, with a cute picture of the Lorax ("Lorax recommended"), plus the following words: earth, green, sustainable, natural, free, and clear. The marketing people are hitting all of my *green* buttons!

The ingredient list is a different matter: water, sodium lauryl sulfate, glycerin, lauramine oxide, caprylyl/myristyl glucoside, magnesium chloride, citric acid, methylisothiazolinone, benzisothiazolinone, essential oils. In this washing liquid, the water, essential oils, and magnesium chloride are natural. By any definition, the manufacturers of this brand are lying when they imply that their dishwashing liquid is natural: sodium lauryl sulfate, lauramine oxide, caprylyl/myristyl glucoside, methylisothiazolinone, and benzisothiazolinone are all synthetic.

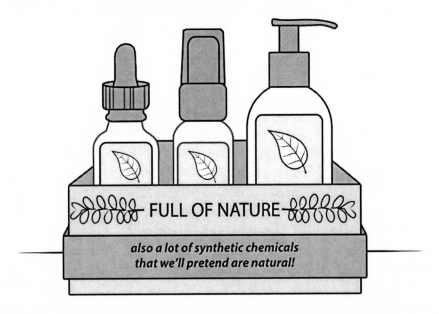

FULL OF NATURE

*also a lot of synthetic chemicals
that we'll pretend are natural!*

There's a popular personal care company from Maine that has a glossary that is hilarious (or depressing, depending on your point of view). Apparently *everything* this company uses is natural! Like propylene glycol, derived from "gas from the earth"; poloxamer 407, obtained from natural gas and oil; glyceryl laurate, from vegetable oils; cocamidopropyl betaine, from coconut oil; coco-glucoside, derived from corn, coconut and palm kernel oils, etc. You get the gist. Their definition of natural is, then, anything that has been derived, by any chemical procedure, from something that exists on earth. In short, they've never encountered anything non-natural. The word "natural" has lost any meaning, except in the commercial, marketing, "feel good without making any effort" sense.

I love botanical extracts; some of them contain valuable chemicals that can benefit you and your skin. I also love some of the synthetic ingredients that are impractical, or too expensive, to obtain from natural sources. Our epidermal growth factor (EGF) is identical to human EGF but is made in a laboratory. It would be impractical and potentially unsafe to use the natural version. To believe this myth is to deny the value of this ingredient - when it is so clearly *beneficial* to our skin.

Myth: Cleanse, tone, moisturize - you *must* have a perfect regimen

Cleaning your skin is important, even if you don't live or work in a polluted city. But what is a toner? Forget about the toners full of alcohol, they will only damage your skin, removing ceramides and oils that the skin needs to perform its function. And what about moisturizer? You need a lot more than that. You should use a cream that helps your skin keep water in and pollutants out. Silicones (the ingredient that gives a *silky feel* to creams and lotions) are perfect for this job, but will do nothing else for your skin and may even slow down absorption of valuable nutrients. So reject silicones and think *nutrition*. Hyaluronic acid, natural active peptides, essential fatty acids, niacinamide and other vitamins will help your skin long-term. And if you're planning to live a long and fruitful life, you need to think long-term.

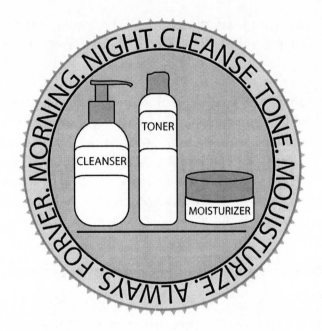

We have been sold this myth because consumers using three products every morning and night is a lucrative situation for skin care companies, but there is no perfect regimen. You don't really need a routine. The environment changes every day, your skin does too, so why stick to a routine that may work one day but not another? Slow down, back off of any regimen and liberate yourself from this myth. You can cleanse in the middle of the day if your skin is feeling too oily. You can spray on a *nourishing* toner anytime day or night. You can have multiple moisturizers that you use for specific reasons, or you can pass on applying a cream if you don't need it. Get to *know* your skin so you can assess its needs. Then you'll be able to choose the product that suits the need as it occurs.

Chapter 4: The chemistry of skin care

An origin myth about proteases

A company has trademarked a fish egg extract. Here's the myth: "Salmon hatchery workers reported that the skin on their hands became soft and felt smooth when they exposed them to the ice-cold hatching fluid from salmon. This was totally unexpected as swollen, red and chapped skin is the normal status of hands after prolonged exposure to cold water. The curious scientists wanted to find the explanation for the smooth skin. They investigated it further and found a protein, which helps the fish embryo getting out of its eggshell. The eggshells are made as a tough, fibrous protein structure, and the fish larva is not able to get out by using mechanical power. They claim this extract helps to digest the eggshell without harming the larva, and thereby allowing the fish to be born. This natural and elegant process combining "rough" digestion of the dead tissue in the eggshell with preservation of the living larvae is also the key in our effective and gentle skin treatment. In order for our skin to regenerate, we need to remove the dead outer layer of our skin."

If you ever had caviar (real or not) you will disagree with the statement that fish eggshells are made of tough, fibrous protein. I have found nothing in the literature to support that assertion (more interesting, proteases are responsible for penetration of the human egg by sperm). What is silly about this "skin care myth"? It assumes that the fish "eggshell" and the exterior layers of our skin have similar proteins. Also, our skin has its own way to remove the dead outer layers.

Now, there's a lot to be said about the benefits of fish eggs for our skin and bodies, like that they're full of nutrients. Feel free to go to the supermarket (Alaskan salmon roe, 8oz for $22.50) and make yourself a nice, nutritive mask using salmon roe. If you don't use the whole jar, the fish eggs will taste really nice on a cracker or rye bread with cream cheese. To make the mask, because the eggs are so tender, you can process them with a food processor or mash them with a fork. Add them to plain, full fat yogurt (full of lactic acid) for a nice, exfoliating mask.

Learn some chemistry to make better choices

Nature is made of chemicals. Many people have forgotten what they learned about nature and chemistry in high school and they get confused when they read on the internet about the dangers of synthetic chemicals. For some, the past may be a golden age, because they don't remember (most were not alive) the time before antibiotics were discovered and vaccines were invented. People who don't spend much time in a natural environment may see nature as a benefactor, a *mother earth* to take care of us and nurture us. That's OK, as long as they don't follow their instincts and try to manufacture a skin care product containing only natural materials. If they don't know any phytochemistry, they may end up making and selling (and people using!) a line based on *Nerium oleander*, a poisonous plant. Or they mix up a lotion without adding a preservative and they find a bad-smelling green and yellow mess after a week. Or how about a serum containing an allergenic plant extract? Or a photosensitizing plant juice? There is no end to the mistakes, many of them lethal, that one can make when using natural ingredients. This is why it's so useful to have the scientists of Skin Actives working for you. What you don't know *can* hurt you!

On the concentration and purity of actives in skin care formulations

You may see many of our actives in some ingredient lists of commercial brand name products. Don't be mistaken by the similarity: there is more to an active than the name. In the industry, plant extracts are usually added as a water/propylene glycol/preservative extract, and the name on the ingredient list will be the same. But at Skin Actives we use powder extracts with the highest available concentration of the active chemical. How can you tell the difference? The difference is often told by color and smell. And though I wish *Centella asiatica* (common names Centella, gotu kola*)* and its asiaticosides were white and smelled like vanilla (think ferulic acid), sadly, they don't. At SAS we decide the concentration to use on the basis of published scientific research, and if our Anti-Aging Cream doesn't smell like roses, so be it.

Label value = negligible amount

"Label value" means that the presence of a name in the ingredient list will make the product more desirable, fashionable, whatever, but please remember that inclusion in the list doesn't necessarily mean that the active is present at a concentration noticeable to your skin, unless, of course, you get your skin care products from Skin Actives Scientific.

Natural smells vs. added fragrances

Some actives have a distinctive odor that some clients may like and others dislike. If they are important actives, we use them anyway. How is it possible that some brands use the same actives we do but their creams smell like a dream? The answer is "label value" (miniscule) concentrations of any active ingredients and the addition of fragrances. The same is true for actives that have strong colors. A yellow active will give its distinctive color to a cream if the concentration is high enough, colors don't just disappear.

We could add fragrances to our products (easily and inexpensively) but prefer to leave whatever is not essential out of our products, giving our clients the option to add fragrances if they want them.

Some examples of chemistry subjects related to skin care

I would not dream of writing a comprehensive book on the chemistry of skin care. It would have to include chemistry (inorganic and organic) plus biochemistry of plants and humans, plus the enumeration of the thousands of ingredients used in skin care.

Fortunately, there are many excellent textbooks and sources for these topics so all I will do here is give you very few examples of how chemistry matters. You don't have to know everything, but it is important that we recognize the complexity of the matter and why we should learn as much as we can about science if we wish to take care of ourselves.

Proteases

Proteases are enzymes that can break down other proteins into small pieces by breaking bonds that link specific amino acids in those proteins. When cooking, have you ever used meat tenderizer? Do you use cold water laundry detergent for your clothes? How about contact lens cleansers? If you answer *yes* to any of these questions, then you have used proteases. Meat tenderizer contains papain. Cold water detergent has subtilisin to break down proteins that stain your clothes. Strong contact lens cleansers also contain subtilisin.

Proteases will not penetrate very far at all, so they are very safe. However, some of us have a tendency to develop allergies: please take into account that many people can become allergic to some proteases, especially papain and subtilisin.

When applied to skin, proteases with the right specificity will hydrolyze the proteins in the most superficial layers of the skin. Our enzymatic peel product is a natural, gentle enzyme "peel" that can be used straight from the bottle. Proteases hydrolyze the proteins, exfoliating dead skin cells and impurities while delivering vitamins and nutrients to the skin. The peel leaves the skin cleansed and silky smooth. Exfoliation will help keep your pores open and free of blackheads and acne letting you show off your new skin, made younger thanks to SAS actives.

Vitamin C

Ascorbic acid

Deficiency of vitamin C results in scurvy (the name "Ascorbic Acid" is derived from the Latin word for scurvy, *scorbutus*), a nasty illness whose easy fix, citrus fruit, eluded pirates and sailors until 1753.

Why is L-ascorbic acid a vitamin? Most animals can make their own vitamin C, but humans can't. Somewhere along the line we lost a crucial enzyme, the L-gulonolactone oxidase, required for the synthesis of L-ascorbic acid, making it an essential nutrient (i.e. we must get it by eating food containing it, or applying the vitamin to our skin).

L-ascorbic acid is important for plants and animals because it works as an antioxidant. More specifically, it is a water soluble antioxidant that works in the cytosol of the cell and the matrix of the orgenelles. Conversely, chemicals with vitamin E activity are lipid (oil) soluble and can work in the lipid region of the cell membranes, including the membrane system of the mitochondria.

There is more to vitamin C than "just" the antioxidant side. In humans, and many animals, ascorbic acid is also a cofactor in the synthesis of carnitine and tyrosine (an amino acid) and it is required for the synthesis of collagen. Collagen is important not only for the skin's appearance, it is also involved in wound-healing and in preventing bleeding from capillaries. Collagen is a protein of complex structure, and the final protein we require is very different from the peptides initially made at the ribosomes. It is composed of a triple helix, which consists of two identical chains and an additional chain that differs slightly in its chemical composition. The amino acid composition of collagen is unusual for proteins with a high content of hydroxyproline. The peptides synthesized in the ribosomes undergo many modifications of their structure before they become collagen; among other modifications, proline (and lysine) residues in the peptides must be hydroxylated in a process catalyzed by enzymes that require ascorbic acid as a cofactor. The many symptoms of scurvy result from the inability of the human body to complete the transformation of the nascent peptides into collagen because of this lack of ascorbic acid. [Incidentally, here you see why it is silly to add hydroxyproline to a skin care product: this amino acid is NOT used in the synthesis of collagen. Protein synthesis requires "plain" proline, and it is only after protein synthesis that the proline residues are hydroxylated.

The "L-" in L-ascorbic acid refers to the position in space of the bonds between atoms. Many molecules have more than one possible structure in space because of the peculiar properties of the carbon atom. These are called asymmetric molecules and the old terminology allows for two mirror forms, L and D (levo and dextro, left and right in Latin, respectively) because of the effect a solution has on polarized light. L-Ascorbic Acid means that the compound's stereochemistry is related to that of the levorotatory enantiomer of glyceraldehyde.

The ascorbic acid we use at Skin Actives Scientific is the L-ascorbic form, but even if you were to get the racemic form (mix of the two stereoisomers) you would still be fine. Both forms have antioxidant activity, and you would get more than enough of the L-form to allow for the enzymatic reactions that require L-ascorbic as a cofactor.

L-ascorbic acid is a water soluble antioxidant, a very important part of the antioxidant system that includes water-soluble and lipid soluble antioxidants and enzymes. In this complex system you will find many of the actives that we use at SAS: alpha-D-tocopherol, tocotrienols and coenzyme Q10 (oil soluble), glutathione (water soluble), superoxide dismutase, and more (see our ROS* Terminator).

How do they work together? When alpha-D-tocopherol donates an electron to "save" a membrane lipid, it becomes oxidized. Ascorbic acid re-reduces the oxidized vitamin E. The oxidized vitamin C is, in turn, re-reduced by glutathione and enzymes. This is the way that the system keeps working, recycling the oxidized antioxidants.

In short, vitamin C is the water soluble antioxidant that will decrease oxidative stress in your skin. This is probably the mechanism by which it inhibits melanogenesis, protects from UVA and UVB radiation, lightens sun spots, and alleviates melasma.

The other effects of ascorbic acid on the skin are probably related to its role as a cofactor in a number of enzymatic reactions. At the biochemical level, L-ascorbic acid promotes synthesis of new collagen, promotes expression of type 1 and type 4 collagens and ascorbic acid transporters, and inhibits the activity of matrix metalloproteinases (enzymes capable of breaking down collagen and elastin). The use of L-ascorbic acid visually improves wrinkles and decreases inflammation.

Vitamin C serums must contain chemicals with vitamin C activity. This may sound obvious, but manufacturers often stretch the truth (naughty and not nice). You will understand this statement if you read the rest of this book.

Dissolved in water, ascorbic acid may be destroyed by the oxygen in the air. This is not a problem when you are taking vitamin C tablets or drinking orange juice, but it becomes a problem for skin care products that need to be on a store shelf for 12 months. Some products that contain ascorbic acid will change color and lose activity within weeks, making them useless.

Organic chemists have been playing with ascorbic acid for a long time, trying to modify its structure to make it more suitable for use in skin care products, while keeping the vitamin C activity intact. Every new chemical derivative requires testing to make sure that the modified molecule still works as vitamin C in aspects relevant to the skin. Because each scientific paper measures activity in a different way, it is important to read the scientific literature (and not just the marketing materials) to make sure that the chemically modified ascorbic acid is still useful.

Some product manufacturers insist that their modified ascorbic acids will be absorbed better than the natural form. This is a bad excuse for chemical modification because L-ascorbic acid is absorbed and used by the skin without any problem.

In the case of Magnesium-L-Ascorbyl-2-Phosphate (MAP), the L-ascorbic acid derivative we use in our Antioxidant and Collagen Serums, MAP releases L-ascorbic acid as it crosses the epidermis. Ascorbyl 2-phosphates, usually formulated as the magnesium salts, are stable in a solution at neutral pH (the phosphate group in the second position of the cyclic ring protects the enediol system of the molecule from oxidation). Ascorbyl phosphate salts are not in themselves antioxidant agents but that is not a problem, because *in vivo* they are converted into L-ascorbic acid (presumably accomplished by the enzyme alkaline phosphatase present in the skin).

MAP is a *good* vitamin C derivative, because it has been shown that it penetrates the skin and in the skin it is converted to L-ascorbic acid. As for the most important question, is MAP an actual vitamin C? MAP has been shown to protect the skin from UV damage and prevent synthesis of melanin, just as L-ascorbic acid does.

MAP offers an extra advantage to some users: for some, the acidity of an L-ascorbic acid solution can sting, but MAP should not. For the formulators, it allows vitamin C to be formulated together with great actives, like epidermal growth factor, which like many other proteins, are unstable in acidic media. This is why in our popular Collagen Serum you will find MAP and not ascorbic acid.

Additionally, we also sell ascorbyl palmitate, another vitamin C derivative. When mixing, in addition to the activity, you have to pay attention to solubility. Ascorbic acid and MAP are water-soluble and therefore perfect for their vitamin C and antioxidant properties required in our Collagen Serum and our Antioxidant Serum. However, sometimes an oil-soluble version of vitamin C is wanted for a special formulation, and for that we turn to ascorbyl palmitate. But it is important to remember that the principal role of vitamin C is as a water-soluble antioxidant.

Glycolic and lactic acids are alpha hydroxyl acids (AHA) frequently used in peels because they are weak acids that will do their job and later be metabolized by the skin. Ascorbic acid is also an AHA and useful for an acidic peel.

Like with all acidic peels, the peel depth is determined by the pH (the lower the pH the more acidic and stronger the peel), determined in turn by the type of acid, its concentration, and whether it was neutralized. Volume applied, time of contact, frequency of application, integrity of skin, skin thickness, skin oiliness, and post-peel care will also affect the results of the peel. AHAs in general will increase the production of collagen, water content of the skin, and synthesis of glycosaminoglycans. Acid peels will increase elastin fibers, volume of the epidermis, and tightening of the superficial skin layers. The lower the pH - the stronger the effect, but there may be more skin irritation as well.

In view of these facts, you can see that vitamin C serums will also work as mild peels, on top of the many benefits of vitamin C, as an enzyme cofactor and antioxidant.

Other ascorbic acid derivatives used in the industry include ascorbyl tetraisopalmitate (tetrahexyldecyl ascorbate), ascorbyl glucoside, and many more to come so that the marketing department can announce "the newest and most powerful vitamin C ever!" In this case, as in many others, new is not necessarily better. We prefer to use MAP and ascorbyl palmitate because they are proven, stable forms of vitamin C.

In short: For a vitamin C serum to actually be a vitamin C serum, the ascorbic acid derivative must be stable (so it is not oxidized before you apply it to your skin), and it must have vitamin C activity *in vivo*. This will require that the derivative is broken down in the skin to produce ascorbic acid and has to display antioxidant activity, melanin inhibition, protection from UV radiation, etc. According to this very common sense definition, some vitamin C serums on the market are probably NOT C serums.

Stereoisomers

Arbutin is one of the many actives we sell as powders, and we also use it as an ingredient in our Skin Brightening Cream. The mechanism of action of arbutin is through the competitive inhibition of the enzyme tyrosinase, a key enzyme in the synthesis of melanin, although it has been suggested that it may also affect other steps in the synthesis and accumulation of melanin.

I have received many emails asking whether the arbutin we use is "alpha or beta". That confused me a bit because the chemical extracted from bearberry (*Artactophylos uva ursi*) is called "arbutin", no alpha or beta, although one of the many synonyms is alpha arbutin. To be sure, I looked it up in the Merck index and I found only arbutin.

After several such emails, I finally realized that the question had to do with the glycosidic bond between the glucose residue and the hydroquinone, but I was still surprised that our clients would be interested in stereochemistry of carbohydrates. The answer to this question was (as usual) in a marketing gimmick.

Arbutin is a relatively simple chemical, with a glucose attached to a hydroquinone. Both hydroquinone and arbutin have skin lightening properties, primarily because they inhibit synthesis of melanin through the competitive inhibition of a crucial enzyme in the pathway. The glucose residue makes a difference: arbutin does not have the side effects that hydroquinone seems to have. Arbutin also has anti-cancer activity on melanoma cells, apparently by regulating expression of the p53 tumor suppressor and cell apoptosis.

Because of the arrangement of atoms in space, there are two ways in which the D-glucose can bind to the hydroquinone, this is why we need the "beta" to describe the structure. The alternative is the "alpha", but bearberry has the biochemical apparatus to make the beta, not the alpha. The alpha stereoisomer can be made in the laboratory, and it is now marketed as "alpha-arbutin", although this name is misleading.

The way the D-glucose binds to the hydroquinone is very likely to make a difference in the behavior of the chemical. For example, the glucose residues in cellulose (think "paper") are bound by beta glycosidic linkages, while the same glucose residues in starch (think "bread") are bound by alpha glycosidic linkages. As you know, you can't make bread with cellulose.

It is disingenuous to suggest that a change in structure from a *beta* glycosidic linkage as in natural arbutin to an *alpha* (like in the novel chemical) is a big enough difference to make the chemical stronger in terms of suppression of pigmentation, while at the same time implying that the novel chemical is as safe as natural arbutin.

Why do we at SAS sell synthetic ascorbic acid derivatives but not the "new" synthetic arbutin? For ascorbic acid, most derivatives are esters of ascorbic acid, which will be quickly transformed by enzymes in the skin to ascorbic acid. In the case of arbutin, the type of sugar and the way it is bound to the hydroquinone represents a qualitative difference, because enzymes capable of using the beta glucosyl will not recognize the alpha glucosyl residue. More and more analogs and derivatives of arbutin may come to the market, e.g. with xylose replacing the glucose but we will not sell them until exhaustive toxicological data become available.

Just like with preservatives, I like to use chemicals that have been proven to be safe and effective. For us at Skin Actives, novelty in a chemical is not an advantage but a problem.

What is the difference between salicin and salicylic acid?

More than one thousand years ago, humans in different continents discovered that the leaves and bark of the willow tree could alleviate aches and fevers. With the advent of modern chemistry, in 1828, salicin, the major salicylate in willow bark, was isolated by Johann Buchner. A few decades later, industrial production of synthetic acetylsalicylic acid, trade name Aspirin, was introduced in Germany by Bayer. In skin care, we use two chemicals of this family: salicin and salicylic acid.

The names of both chemicals originate in from the Latin "Salix", willow tree, from the bark of which the substance used to be obtained. The salts and esters of salicylic acid are known as salicylates, and acetylsalicylic acid, a.k.a. aspirin, is one of them.

Salicylic acid belongs to a diverse group of plant phenolics, compounds with an aromatic ring bearing a hydroxyl group or a derivative. These ubiquitous chemicals are present in plants for reasons that have nothing to do with human headaches, but are related to the regulation of plant physiology and resistance to pathogens.

It is true that salicylic acid is naturally present in many plants, but plants are not the usual source of the salicylic acid used in skin care. Salicylic acid is present at very low concentrations in plants, where it fulfills the role of a hormone and it would be terribly expensive to extract it from plants. The salicylic acid we use is synthesized in laboratories using organic chemistry methods, not that this matters at all: synthetic and natural salicylic acid are indistinguishable from each other.

Salicylic Acid

Salicylic acid has antibacterial keratolytic, anti-inflammatory activities and is used in skin care to penetrate the skin in a suitable solvent (alcohol, petrolatum) where it will exert its anti-inflammatory and antibacterial effect. Salicylic acid works by facilitating the shedding of the cells of the epidermis, opening clogged pores and preventing acne, but at high concentrations it can cause chemical burns like other acids.

Salicin

Salicin is an alcoholic β-glucoside. In the human body the molecule is broken and glucose and salicylic alcohol are metabolized separately. By oxidizing the alcohol function the aromatic part finally is metabolized to salicylic acid. The differences in chemical structure make salicin "mild" or non-irritating to the skin.

In skin care, salicin and salicylic acid have different applications. The milder, non-irritating salicin, is present in our acne and anti-inflammatory products.

Q. Why is salicylic acid called "beta hydroxy?"

A. This weak acid is called beta hydroxyl acid in the skin care industry "just because". No excuse whatsoever and no connection to the "beta hydroxyl" in chemistry.

Q. What is the main difference between salicylic acid and alpha hydroxy acids like lactic acid?

A. They are completely different in their chemical structure, resulting in completely different solubilities.

Q. What is the mechanism of the anti-inflammatory effect of salicylates?

A. Salicylic acid has been shown to suppress the activity of cyclooxygenase (COX), an enzyme that is responsible for the production of pro-inflammatory mediators such as the prostaglandins. It does this by suppression of the expression of the enzyme.

Fatty acids

A fatty acid (example: palmitic acid) has a carboxylic acid attached to a long hydrocarbon chain. Fatty acids are used as a major source of energy during metabolism and as a starting point for the synthesis of phospholipids, the main category of lipid molecules used to construct biological membranes (generally composed of two fatty acids linked through glycerol phosphate to one of a variety of polar groups).

The chemical structure makes the function possible. Stearic acid cannot do what linoleic acid can.

Fatty acids can differ in:

1. Number of carbon in the chain.
2. Number and carbon position of the double (unsaturated) bond (the ω refers to the position of the double bond relative to the #1 carbon in the chain).
3. Configuration of the unsaturated bond (cis vs. trans). A "cis" bond bends the chain in space and is very important for the fluidity of cell membranes.

Note: "trans" bonds are not usually found in nature but in synthetic, hydrogenated fats. Whose idea was it to hydrogenate vegetable oils to make margarine? And who decided that they were healthier than butter?

An essential fatty acid is one that humans and other animals must obtain from food because the body requires them for good health. We cannot synthesize them because we don't have the enzymes (desaturases 12 and 15) required to synthesize them from the saturated fatty acid stearic acid.

Only two fatty acids are known to be essential for humans: alpha-linolenic acid (an omega-3 fatty acid) and linoleic acid (an omega-6 fatty acid).

Some other fatty acids are sometimes classified as "conditionally essential", meaning that they can become essential under some developmental or disease conditions; examples include docosahexaenoic acid (an omega-3 fatty acid) and gamma-linolenic acid (an omega-6 fatty acid). At SAS we use a variety of plant and algae fatty acids to ensure that our skin has a good supply of both essential and conditional essential fatty acids.

Figure: linoleic acid, an essential fatty acid abundant in pitaya oil. Note the position of the double bonds relative to the omega Carbon 1).

Cell membranes are crucial to health. Deficiency in essential fatty acids shows as dermatitis.

Fatty acids in general are central to the use of energy in the skin, required to make new skin and maintain function and health.

Lectins and the skin

The first human lectin was identified in 1974, but the work on skin lectin receptors lags well behind that on receptors present in other human organs. There is a receptor lectin in fibroblasts and keratinocytes that recognizes rhamnose (a methyl pentose) not synthesized by humans. From the point of view of skin aging, an issue so dear to the skin care industry (including us at SAS!), it is known that applying rhamnose containing glycans to the skin stimulates cell proliferation, decreases elastase-type activity, stimulates collagen biosynthesis, and protects hyaluronan against free radical mediated degradation. This is a very useful effect, even if we don't know what the primary function of this receptor lectin is. Based on what we know about lectin receptors, we can hypothesize that they have something to do with the beneficial bacteria that live on our skin, but the receptor could also be just an evolutionary leftover. Living organisms, and even viruses, possess sophisticated enzymatic systems devoted to making the glycans, and also the lectins that recognize them.

People with skin conditions characterized by excessive cell division, like psoriasis, should avoid glycans that promote cell division. However, glycans that modulate the immune response, like fucoidans and yeast beta glucans, should be fine.

Lectins may be implicated in allergy: galectin-3 is highly expressed in epithelial cells, including keratinocytes, and is involved in the pathogenesis of inflammatory skin diseases by affecting the functions of immune cells. For example, galectin-3 can contribute to atopic dermatitis and may also be involved in the development of contact hypersensitivity by regulating migration of antigen presenting cells. Human milk contains non-digestible oligosaccharides and modulates allergy, another connection to the role of glycans in allergy.

References:

Faury G, Ruszova E, Molinari J, Mariko B, Raveaud S, Velebny V, Robert L. (2008) The alpha-1-rhamnose recognizing lectin site of human dermal fibrolasts functions as a signal transducer. Modulation of Ca++ fluxes and gene expression. Biochim.Biophys.Acta. 2008. pp. 1388-1394.

Larsen, Larissa, Chen, Huan-Yuan; Saegusa, Jun, Liu, Fu-Tong (2011) Galectin-3 and the skin. J Dermatological Science, 64: 85-91.

Oh JH, Kim YK, Jung JY, Shin JE, Chung JH.(2011) Changes in glycosaminoglycans and related proteoglycans in intrinsically aged human skin in vivo. Experimental Dermatology. 20:454-6

Sharon, N. and Lis H. (2004) History of lectins: from hemagglutinins to biological recognition molecules, in Glycobiology, 14: 53R–62R.

Ceramides

Ceramides consist of a long-chain or sphingoid base linked to a fatty acid via an amide bond.

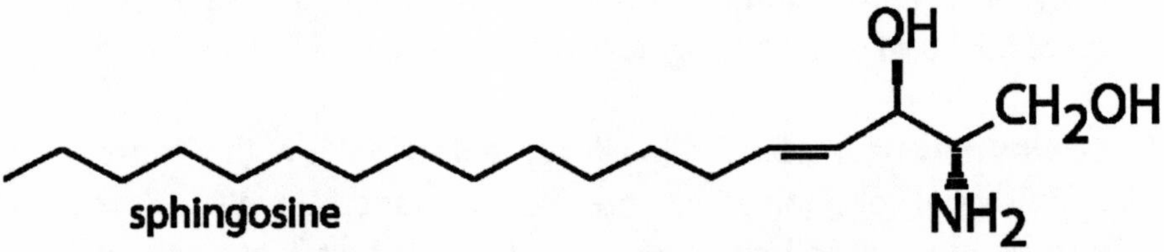

Sphingosine

R.CHOH.CH.CH2OH
|
NHOC.R

ceramide

Ceramide, with sphingosine bound to a fatty acid via an amide

Ceramides are present at low concentration in plants and animals, so there isn't a good source of natural ceramides for use in the industry. Extraction of a rare chemical from a plant requires laborious processes and the resulting ingredients are terribly expensive. Another source of ceramides, the central nervous system, is not suitable for epidemiological reasons. For this reason, the ceramides used in skin care are synthetic. This is not a problem because ceramides in skin have structural roles that can be filled by many chemicals.

The scientific nomenclature for ceramides is simple enough: it combines the names for fatty acids and long-chain bases to denote the molecular species of ceramides, e.g. N-palmitoyl-sphingosine is d18:1-16:0.

For ceramides, the INCI (International nomenclature for cosmetic ingredients) nomenclature is not helpful. For the synthetic ceramide caproyl sphingosine (about $25,000 per gram, for comparison, the price of pure gold is around $40 per gram), with CAS# 100403-19-8, several INCI names are used: Ceramide 5, ceramide 4, ceramide 3, ceramide 2, ceramide 1, ceramide 1A, ceramide 6, ceramide 6II, etc.

A typical ingredient list of a ceramide mix used in the industry will read as follows: Ceramide 3 (and) Ceramide 6 (and) Ceramide I (and) Phytosphingosine (and) Cholesterol (and) Sodium Lauroyl Lactylate (and) Carbomer (and) Xanthan Gum.

Even with additives, this ingredient still costs several thousand dollars per Kg. The INCI name for the ceramide is "ceramide E", and CAS No is 153967-07-8. Synonyms: Cetyl-PG Hydroxyethyl Palmitamide.

If you look at the chemical formula below, you will see that this is not strictly a ceramide, thus its name "pseudoceramide". Pseudoceramides were created to solve the problem created by topical steroids, a medication used for serious inflammatory illnesses; when used long term corticosteroids affect the skin in negative ways. Pseudoceramides are capable of forming lamellar structures like those ceramides form; they will restore the skin barrier, decreasing water loss in skin damaged by corticosteroid use.

Ceramide E (chemical name Cetyl-PG Hydroxyethyl Palmitamide)

Ceramides are an important part of what makes the epidermis a good barrier against water loss. They form part of the "cement" that together with flattened, a-nucleated cells (corneocytes) make the cornified layer (stratum corneum, SC) of the epidermis. The SC is central to the role of skin as a barrier against water loss, bacterial and fungal attacks, and penetration of anything foreign to the skin.

The most external layer is the stratum corneum, preventing water loss and entry of noxious substances. How is the stratum corneum formed? In the layer below, keratinocytes are losing their nuclei and releasing polar lipids that will be transformed into ceramides and free fatty acids.

The SC consists of corneocytes, flattened cells that have lost their nuclei, imbedded in a lipid mixture consisting mainly of a lamellar structure of ceramides, cholesterol, and free fatty acids. Insufficient lipids or lipids in the "wrong" ratio (because some were lost or there were not enough in the first place) can result in an increased water loss and/or increased penetration of harmful substances from the environment causing skin dryness and skin sensitivity

Now, we can make a big thing of this and say that we need to plaster the skin with topically applied ceramides in order to improve the barrier, but by the time ceramides are deposited in the epidermis it is a bit too late to change much. In my opinion, the time to work on a good stratum corneum is long before it has been formed: provide your live skin cells with the polar lipids they will use later on to make ceramides. As for the fundamental role of the stratum corneum, the corner stone of the skin barrier, at this late stage other actives may do just as well.

What is collagen?

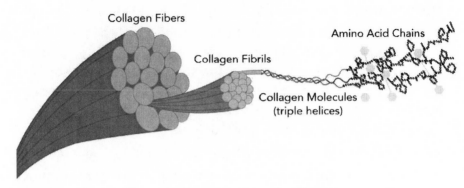

Collagen Fibers

Amino Acid Chains

Collagen Fibrils

Collagen Molecules
(triple helices)

The complex structure of collagen

Collagen fibers give the skin resistance to strain and traction. Collagen constitutes about 70% of skin mass, but total collagen decreases about 1% per year. It may look like a small decline, but as such a major component of the skin it will affect skin volume and its physical properties. Also, aging changes collagen structure. What was an organized pattern in young skin, becomes an assembly of disorganized bundles of thick fibrils in older skin. It is not only quantity; it is also quality.

We know that aging decreases skin thickness and elasticity, and it is likely that collagen is a good part of the solution. If we care about slowing down and reversing skin aging, we should care about collagen too. Because collagen is such a major constituent of the skin, the objective should be to stimulate its synthesis, and preserve the collagen protein in an active, organized structure.

Chemically, we want to prevent glycation, the attachment of sugar moieties to the protein amino acids, a modification that affects protein function. The fibroblasts are the main cells in the dermis. They specialize in producing two types of proteins, collagen and elastin, which are a major part of the extra-cellular matrix.

Collagen is synthesized by fibroblasts, initially as procollagen alpha chains on membrane-bound ribosomes. The alpha chains then interact to form a triple-helical molecule after hydroxylation of proline and lysine amino acids. Stability is further enhanced by disulfide cross-linking. The procollagen is then packaged into secretory vesicles that move to the cell surface. At the cell membrane, procollagen peptidases cleave the procollagen into collagen.

Collagen is a structural, long-lived protein. Even if synthesis decreases, the total content may not decrease, it will depend on how much collagen was hydrolyzed by protease action. Proteolysis is not bad in itself, it is good for the skin to eliminate proteins whose structure and properties have been modified beyond usefulness.

Skin aging means, mostly, photoaging. To see the net effect of UV on skin aging, compare the outside of your arm with the underside, a skin area you don't usually expose to the sun. UV radiation increases the synthesis of proteases, including collagenase, and this is likely to be a reason why collagen decreases after UV irradiation. Natural aging decreases collagen synthesis and increases the expression of matrix metalloproteinases, whereas photoaging results in an increase of collagen synthesis and greater matrix metalloproteinase expression in human skin in vivo. Thus, the balance between collagen synthesis and degradation leading to collagen deficiency is different in photoaged and naturally aged skin. A good part of the changes in collagen related to aging seem to be associated with decreased levels of estrogen.

Standardized phytochemicals

Not all plant extracts are the same. Some plant extracts are beneficial and this is because there are some useful chemicals in the mix of hundreds present in the extract. As phytochemistry progresses, it is possible to identify the beneficial chemicals.

What are the advantages of identification of the active chemical? Once you know what works in that mix, it is possible to separate the useful chemical from the rest by using a variety of purification methods. Step by step, you get the active chemical more and more pure. This process is costly but has advantages: it is less likely to have negative effects from other, non beneficial chemicals that accompany the good one in the total extract, and the pure chemical may be more pleasing and more compatible with the carrier than the initial extract.

Sometimes, a plant contains so many beneficial chemicals that it does not make sense to purify one of them. This is the case with our sea kelp extract ferment which supplies a complete nutrient medium and moisturizes skin and scalp. The substrate for fermentation is kelp, a sea macroalgae (Phaeophyta). Fermentation makes the cell contents of these algae readily available to our skin and scalp. This maximizes its moisturizing properties, as well as making nutrients available that are required by the skin. The ferment also has a calming, anti-itch activity.

The bioferment is rich in fucoidan, caragenaan, algin, minerals, and many active chemicals. It also provides minerals like iodine, copper, molybdate, magnesium, and others required as cofactors in enzymatic reactions of lipid metabolism and energy conversion. Fucoxanthin is a pigment present in Phaeophyta (brown algae) that may protect skin from photo-aging caused by UV. Fucoidans are sulfated polysaccharides with structures that depend on the plant source and growing conditions. Applied to the skin, fucoidan will increase the density of collagen bundles, decrease activity of proteases (enzymes that break down dermal proteins), increase scavenging of free radicals, and increase cell proliferation. These effects would be mediated through increased expression of ß1-integrin and may also help with wound healing. In addition to assisting in collagen synthesis, fucoidan inhibits the replication of many viruses, including herpes, human cytomegalovirus, HIV-1, and others.

Faking the science

I was excited when I watched a BBC program on glycobiology and how a global cosmetic brand was investing in research aimed at designing new products. At that time, their new product from the most luxurious brand of their many brands was an anti-aging line with the addition of saffron.

Now I see that my dear BBC was being used as a vehicle for unpaid advertising. The research done by the global corporation was just for show. The "new" cream was a very old formulation, rich in petrolatum and mineral oil, but now with a hint of saffron. But advertising pays, because this product was the talk of the town in New York, at least for a while. At $400 a jar of what is essentially a supermarket brand quality cream, you may want to know what is going on.

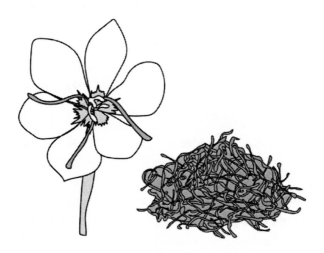

Saffron - the secret ingredient of an excellent Spanish paella, is just OK for skin care.

This is the ingredient list for the "anti-aging" cream: water, glycerin, hydrogenated polyisobutene, mineral oil, butylene glycol, cyclohexasiloxane, cetyl alcohol, glyceryl stearate, corn germ oil, palm oil, PEG 100-stearate, beeswax, myristyl myristate, saffron, apricot kernel oil, corn oil, PEG-14M, argan oil, microcrystalline wax, paraffin, sorbitan tristearate, sorbitol, glyceril acrylate/acrylic acid copolymer, dimethyl isosorbide, isohexadecane, sodium hydroxide, 2-oleamido-1,3-octadecaniol, adenosine, disodium EDTA, propylene glycol, hydrolyzed soy protein, hydroxypropyl tetrahydropropyrantriol, capryloyl salicylic acid, passion flower seed oil, maltitol, xanthan gum, chestnut seed extract, polysorbate 80, acrylamide/sodium acryloyldimethyltaurate copolymer, octyldodecanol, rice bran oil, tocopherol, pentraerithrytil tetra-di-butyl hydroxycinnamate, phenoxyethanol, chlorphenesin, red 4, yellow 5, geraniol, alpha isomethylionone, limonene, citronellol, benzyl alcohol, fragrance.

In short, plenty of fragrances, artificial colorants (why, if saffron has that beautiful color?), occlusive petroleum jelly, wax, mineral oil and little else. The advertising campaign is focused on a miniscule part of an ingredient present in miniscule amounts: saffron. What's so special about saffron? It is an essential spice for paella. It also contains crocin, a carotenoid, which gives saffron its beautiful color and it has antioxidant activity. Other chemical components of saffron like safranal and picrocin contribute to its aroma and characteristic taste.

Let me be clear: I am not criticizing the use of saffron by this large cosmetics company. SAS clients know how much we appreciate carotenoids: astaxanthin is present in almost all of our products. Some carotenoids (alpha carotene, beta carotene) can be used by humans to make vitamin A, another of our favorite ingredients (as retinyl acetate). We also use lutein, fucoxanthin, and lycopene. Carotenoids are good for our health and they're beautiful because of their color.

We at SAS are not planning to sell saffron but you can get some in your supermarket; you can buy the intact saffron or the powder. Just add some to your European Base Cream and you will have your own high quality version without paying silly prices for FD&C Yellow 5 (Trisodium 1-(4-sulfonatophenyl)-4-(4-sulfonatophenylazo)-5-pyrazolone-3-carboxylate) and Red 4 (Disodium 3-[(2,4-Dimethyl-5-sulfonatophenyl) hydrazinylidene]-4-oxonaphthalene-1-sulfonate). With the rest of the saffron, make a great paella.

Chapter 5: Different: the Skin Actives Scientific way

Myth: Expensive skin care products are better

People may be surprised to learn that many women, instead of being deterred by high prices, are encouraged by them. The attitude seems to be "I deserve it" and "If it's expensive, it must be better".

I can sympathize with the "I deserve it" point of view. I love pretty things and I am attracted to the gorgeous containers used by the most expensive lines, and when I am blue I feel like something pretty and expensive may help. BUT, there is a catch. Women buying the most expensive products may be buying bad products, because there is a surprising lack of correlation between the price of a product and the quality of what is inside that jar. Moreover, by buying a bad product you are not using a good product, so you are actually depriving your skin of what it needs, letting it age faster than it should. If you have the money, go ahead BUT, unless the product is good (besides being expensive) this will be bad for you because it will be a wasted opportunity to do something useful for your skin.

Incidentally, the abundance of products with French sounding names is sad. In France people prefer English sounding names!

Spending money makes us feel rich, even if we have to borrow money to pay for the $1,200 bottle of anti-aging cream; but it should make us feel silly. Get SAS, save money and feel clever, because you are getting the best.

Do it yourself

I get many emails asking me how to emulate a specific product, and after I go through the ingredient list and cross out the ingredients that have to do with texture and fragrance, I am often left with *nothing*. Then I wonder whether the prospective client really likes the product or whether they're only responding to advertising. The advertised product is *expensive* so it must be *good*, right? No, not really.

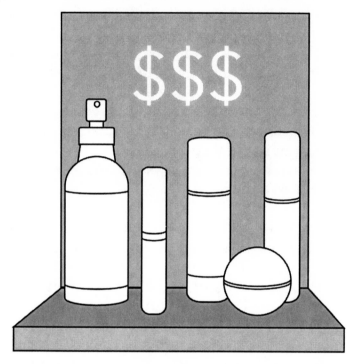

After discussing the ingredient lists of so many expensive brand products, it becomes clear why many people prefer to go the *DIY* way. I hope people are doing this for the right reasons. For a key example, preservatives are *essential* to keeping any skin care product safe, *unless* it will be refrigerated and used within a week of mixing or it has no water in it. Water is a breeding ground for bacteria and as such, preservatives are vital. I am all for saving money, but I hope the main reason someone decides to go DIY is to get the best possible skin care products. We believe you can do both: save money *and* use the very best.

DIY or fancy store skin care?

When we started Skin Actives Scientific, our idea was to provide the active ingredients that would allow our clients to copy the actions of their favorite skin care products and possibly improve on them in their own skin care formulations. What were their reasons to opt out of fancy store skin care? Usually the prices, but also the idea of adding a good active, like coenzyme Q10, at a higher concentration more likely to help the skin. Spending time mixing ingredients was not attractive to some clients, especially when dealing with actives that were hard to dissolve. When many clients asked for base serums and creams so that they would not have to deal with formulation, I realized that our focus should change from selling ingredients to making finished products.

Our first step was putting together kits of actives that went well together and a cream to dissolve them in. Serums followed and soon I was in a position to say, without blushing, that our own products were better than anything sold in department stores. We improved on each formulation, eventually producing creams with each active at optimal concentration. We left out fragrances, colorants, and unnecessary ingredients and we chose simple packaging so that our ready-mixed products end up costing the client less than if they made them from scratch.

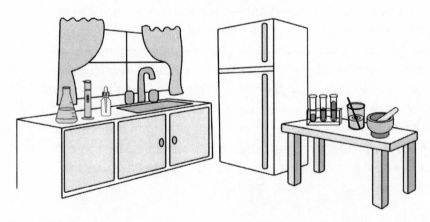

If you have a skin care problem, try the SAS product designed to address your need or you can start with a base cream suitable for your skin (Canvas or European) and add the actives you really want. You can personalize any product; add emolliency with a hint of rosehip oil or for fragrance, add a drop of essential oil or your favorite perfume.

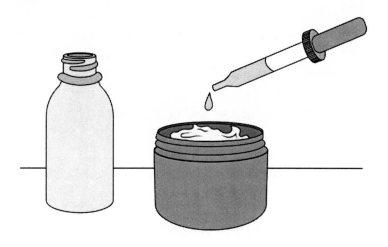

Deceptive labeling can increase consumer risk for DIY adepts

A cream was introduced to the market containing alpha hydroxyl acids with *the highest possible percentage*. That high percentage is what is then used to attract buyers in the DIY camp. It is unlikely that a DIY practitioner will have a good understanding of pH, acidity, buffers and other related subjects that I studied in college and practiced daily in the laboratory for decades. So what happens when a consumer likes a cream that, according to its label, *contains 20% glycolic acid*? They believe it; they feel that the purchase will yield a positive result. They don't notice that on the label the ingredient immediately after glycolic acid is sodium hydroxide, indicating that the main component in that cream is not really glycolic acid as an acid but its *salt*. What the manufacturers of the cream have done is add a lot of glycolic acid so that they could say *our cream contains 20%!!!! and 20% is a lot more than 10%!!!!*. Then they neutralized the acid with a base like sodium hydroxide so that the product will not be dangerous. By neutralizing the acid, they keep the skin safe - but they have been deceptive to their customers.

If a DIY fan decides to save money and buy glycolic acid somewhere, they may or may not know that a product with 20% glycolic acid can burn your skin. Unless you are familiar with acids, bases, buffers and the politics of skin care labeling, please leave that side of things to the experts. What you don't know can hurt you - it can even burn your skin.

A commonly asked question

Question: "I'm 60 years of age, and have noticed that my skin has really begun to show the signs of aging: creases, sun spots, wrinkles, and dullness. Ugh! If I wanted to make my own products, what would you recommend I purchase?"

Answer: To get immediate results and feel better about your skin, massage a few ascorbic acid crystals on damp skin, rinse after a few minutes. You will love the way your skin looks and feels after this. For long term results, I would suggest some ready-mixed products. If you like the way your skin improves (and it will, for sure) you can start mixing your own products using the actives in the products that work. Why take this route? It's the easiest and least expensive, and it'll give you great results. If I give you a long list of actives to mix, you will have to spend more money and if your first attempts to *mix your own* fail, you will lose patience and give up. So, to start, use Vitamin A Cream at night and Collagen Serum both day and night. And if your skin is dry, use Dream Cream or ELS Serum. For sun spots, use UV Repair Cream.

If you decide to go the DIY route: solubility data are available only for water (and sometimes acetone, or ethanol - solvents used in the lab). For everything else you have to *test* solubility, using small amounts of base and active. Please don't forget to add preservative to anything that contains water, otherwise you could catch a nasty infection.

The take-home message for DIY: there is no magic formula. How many actives and how much you can *get in* will depend on the base you use, the solubility of the different actives in that base and the interaction between actives. Start by writing down what you want from the mix, then choose the actives that can do the job, and pick the base most capable of solubilizing the actives. You may need several mixes to accommodate all the actives. Then you will have to test for the solubility of each active, by adding small amounts and mixing.

What Skin Actives Scientific can do for DIY fans

We offer all the actives we know are worth using at near 100% for pure chemicals and at the highest concentration of the active chemicals for natural extracts (like >98% for EGCG). We also have specialty proteins, including antioxidant enzymes and pure growth factors.

If we don't sell an active you want, write to us! We will search the scientific literature to see whether there is research showing that the active is safe and effective; if it is we will acquire it for our clients. This was what happened with nobiletin, an active suggested to us by a client.

Elle magazine has covered our approach by comparing the famous (and hyper expensive) cream from the ocean (but they say it in French) with our Skin Actives Formulation for Beginner's kit. The most notable difference is in the price, and the concentration of actives in the Skin Actives DIY kit will be higher. Also, if you don't like fragrances you don't have to use them (for people with sensitive skin, fragrance in products can cause redness and irritation). Though Elle compared our beginner's kit with the famous brand and called it "faking it", we would prefer *emulating*, as in "match or surpass, typically by imitation".

Some good and some bad reasons to try DIY

Good

1) You'll be able to adapt skin care products to your own needs. You can adjust the emolliency and texture of your cream or lotion. You can add actives for your specific needs and even add your favorite fragrance or avoid fragrances completely.

2) You can use actives at the right concentrations. Many luxury products mention actives in their ingredient labels, but when dozens of items are listed, how can you tell that the one you want was added at the right concentration? This is especially true for actives that aren't white or don't smell nice.

3) You are empowered to imitate a product you love that might be terribly expensive. We don't sing to the bacteria fermenting the sea kelp like a popular brand says they do, so you can get a fantastic cream with kelp bioferment without emptying your bank account.

Don't do DIY if...

1) You're trying to avoid preservatives. If you are using ingredients that bacteria and mold love (like hyaluronic acid, ascorbic acid and practically everything else) your products are just as yummy for bugs as those you will find on the shelves of Macy's. Bacteria and mold spores are in our environment and will start multiplying and using the ingredients in your mix as energy and carbon sources, as soon as you add water. You will not see them unless you have a microscope at home, but believe me, they are there. Among the bacteria, there may be some dangerous ones, and you may end up with an eye infection or something equally nasty.

2) You want to copy expensive products that are not worth copying. Please don't mistake the prices of skin care products as an index of their quality and efficacy, because most of the cost of *luxury* skin care goes to marketing and packaging, and not to the formulation.

3) You're looking for the highest concentration of an active you can get. Most actives will do no harm if you use them at very high concentrations. Likely all that will happen is that you will waste some money, but a few actives at high concentrations, like copper peptides, can hurt your skin. Our skin needs copper at minute concentrations, so when your skin care product is a nice blue because you added lots of copper, expect *loss* of skin elasticity instead of an improvement.

4) You're hoping to get stronger "at home" chemical peels. *Please* don't think that you can make your own acid peel at home. You can certainly prepare an acid solution, but you have no way to make it safely. If you're trying to imitate an alpha hydroxy acid product on the market, please take into account that these products tend to be heavily buffered so that a high concentration can be advertised. Using the percentage of acid stated on the label, unbuffered, may end up causing you a chemical burn. I've answered so many emails of people who ended up in exactly that situation.

Tips for the DIY beginner

1) Use our forum and blog for DIY ideas. Read our DIY FAQ page.

2) Remember that the laws of nature apply. You won't be able to dissolve a water soluble chemical in oil and vice versa. Alcohol will still denature proteins. You can't dissolve more ascorbic acid in water than the chemical structures of water and ascorbic acid will allow. Bacteria and mold will be everywhere.

3) Look at our website to find actives that can help with your specific skin issue.

4) Start simple and easy, and think of what you wish to achieve and avoid in terms of a regimen. The simplest way is to use our beginner's kit, or just add an active you want to try to one of our base creams.

5) Intuition will not replace knowledge. Don't underestimate the expertise required to make a safe, effective skin care product. Read about pH, emulsions, microbiology, and use reputable sources or a good textbook.

The most frequently asked questions about DIY

Do I need to add a preservative to my DIY serum? Answer: Yes, unless you work in very clean conditions, which you should do anyway. Refrigerate your mix and use it within a week. Otherwise, be aware that you'll be sharing your actives with millions of organisms that are as hungry as your skin. This is true for any mix containing water, be it a cream, lotion, or serum.

Do you sell the preservative grapefruit seed extract? Answer: No, because an extract of grapefruit seed would not prevent the growth of bacteria or mold. The preservative mixes called by this name are not extracts, but plant material converted chemically into some strong preservatives that are *not* natural or safe. It has been shown in many scientific publications that commercial grapefruit seed extracts are not what they say they are, because they have been adulterated with synthetic antimicrobial chemicals such as benzethonium chloride, 1,3,5-trimethoxybenzene, benzalkonium chloride, 4-hydroxybenzoic acid esters and more.

What not to mix?

This is probably one of the most frequent questions arriving in my email inbox and to the forum. My answer is that I know of only a few rules, the rest is trial and error. Even the few rules I know of and apply in our own products aren't a matter of life and death, except for our specialty proteins, which will likely *die* (denature) under extreme pH conditions (very acidic or very alkaline).

I also know that ascorbic acid derivatives can do strange things in the presence of metals like copper or iron, so I tell clients to use distilled water to dissolve ascorbic acid. On the other hand, using ascorbic acid crystals as an exfoliator after a shower is unlikely to do any harm in a matter of minutes or at the very high ascorbic acid concentrations we are using. In short, what matters in theory is unlikely to matter much in practice. Conversely, fear can ruin our quality of life. I don't like fear, which these days the internet seems to spread faster than ever, at a time when we, in economically advanced countries such as ours, are reaching our ninetieth birthdays and further.

Many mixtures of actives will turn into an ugly mess, so start with small quantities. If you mess up, don't throw away the mess. The actives are still in there, even if they precipitated, or liquefied the cream or whatever may have happened. Try mixing a little bit of the *mess* with a body lotion, or maybe with water and see what happens. If something works, write it down while you still remember what you did! And visit our forum, our members have a lot of collective experience and they can help.

Chapter 6: Skin, the environment, and oxidation

Myth: Your skin needs extra oxygen

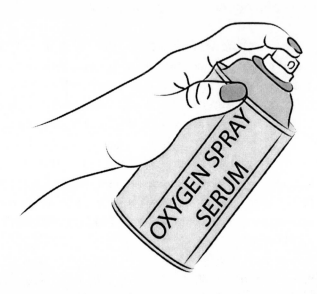

No, your skin doesn't need extra oxygen. Skin gets more than enough oxygen from the air and through the blood vessels that irrigate the dermis. In fact, your skin gets *too much* oxygen, and oxygen is partly to blame for aging skin. The "excess" does not result in more energy, because our blood and mitochondria are saturated with oxygen (they have as much as they need to carry on their functions) but the extra free radicals will age the skin, increase mutations in our cells' DNA and break down the lipids in the cell membranes. So if anybody invites you to an oxygen bar, run in the opposite direction. If somebody else wants to sell you a cream made with hemoglobin (read: cow's blood) tell them that dead, yucky protein cannot carry oxygen and even if it could, that oxygen would do nothing good for your skin.

Our skin and the environment

The role of our skin is to separate us from the environment. Our body's composition on the inside is so different from the outside that we need our skin in order for the body to function properly. When our skin does not function as it should, the consequences are felt as pain, infection, and damage to the body.

Our skin protects us in many different ways: it prevents water loss, protects us from radiation and guards us from infection. Our skin is also a great communicator - bringing us useful information about the environment through our sense of touch and our perception of pain. But the protection our skin provides doesn't come for free; a lifetime of defense can lead to scars, wrinkles and hyperpigmentation. With all of the damage that will occur naturally - it's surprising that anyone would want to make it worse by smoking, tanning, or getting laser treatments. There are also a lot of products out there that I call *skin care from hell* - to be avoided at all costs for the long-term health of your skin.

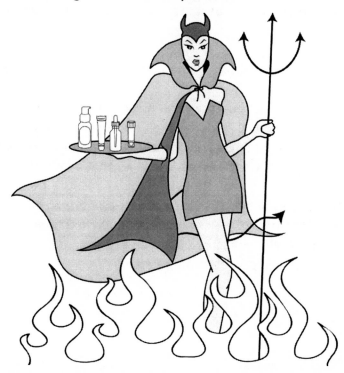

The skin barrier

Our skin acts as a protector against water loss and physical, chemical, and biological attack. To perform its protective task, the skin must have a resistant barrier. This barrier is provided by the *horny layer* or *stratum corneum*, the outermost layer of the epidermis. An insufficient formation or excess loss of skin lipids can result in an increased water loss and increased penetration of harmful compounds from the environment, both of which often cause skin dryness and skin sensitivity.

We are mostly water, and the air is relatively dry; our bodies could not function if we lost too much water to the air, so our skin has to be relatively impermeable to water. Also, our cells must be protected from microbes that would be only too happy to multiply inside us; our skin has to be impermeable to spores, bacteria, and more.

Does the skin do its job? Yes, when it's healthy, thanks to the intricate structure of the horny layer, a compact brick wall-like layer made of corneocytes (mature keratinocytes that lost their organelles) and special lipids in which the corneocytes are the *bricks* and the intercellular lipids (which include ceramides) and proteins are the *mortar*. This is the protective layer that allows the rest of the skin to do its job, even though it is *dead* because the cells are not metabolically active. Preventing trans-epidermal, or through-the-skin, water loss (TEWL) is one of the main functions of the horny layer. TEWL is measured using an instrument that can determine water vapor loss from the skin.

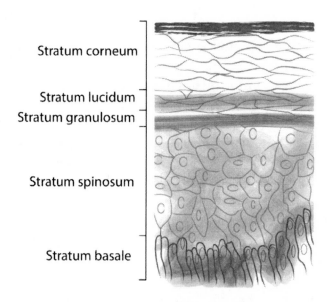

Stratum corneum

Stratum lucidum
Stratum granulosum

Stratum spinosum

Stratum basale

Skin cells change shape and structure to form the different layers of the skin. Cornified cells (corneocytes) are dead cells, but together they make a layer (horny layer, stratum corneum in Latin) that prevents water loss and the entry of microbes.

The upper layer is rich in *natural moisturizing factor* (NMF), a mixture of amino acids and derivatives with great binding capacity for water. NMF keeps the skin hydrated, but can be lost with frequent washing. It is worth noting that many ingredients used in the skin care industry, like ceramides and sodium PCA, are chosen from those present naturally in the skin. It makes sense to start skin care by avoiding routines that remove these natural ingredients. Some people complain of skin sensitivity and dryness while using peels and strong detergents in a misguided effort to keep their skin and pores "clean".

Sun damage, detergents, and mistreatment can lead the skin to lose its impermeability to water. You can help keep the skin barrier intact by using skin care products containing actives that will act as replacements for chemicals that are present naturally in healthy skin like linoleic acid, ceramides, sodium PCA, and others. The chemical structure does not need to be identical, as long as they can do a good job, for example the ceramides present naturally in the skin can be substituted by other waxy lipids.

Besides using chemicals that mimic those used by the skin to keep its barrier properties intact, sometimes it helps to cover the skin with products that will keep it from losing water. Mineral oil, petrolatum, and lanolin will help while the skin is repairing itself and incapable of doing its job properly. Some forums have tried to discredit these ingredients (petroleum derived, etc.) but they are still used in very expensive skin care products in order to achieve the right texture.

An interesting fact is that older skin is a better barrier than you would expect, despite a significant decline in nutrients reaching it. The way this is achieved is by the old corneocytes staying put longer, so you get more layers of dead cells, partly compensating for the decrease in lipids. For this reason, sodium lauryl sulfate, the king of surfactants (detergent chemicals that interact with water and lipids), and much loved because it can form large bubbles, does not induce water loss from older skin as much as it does from younger skin. Interesting, isn't it? Our skin gets older and uglier but it still manages to do its job to some extent. Let's be nicer to it - we can start by protecting it from the sun.

Sunlight is more than what we see

Ultraviolet light is classified into three categories: UVA (long wave, black light, 315 to 400 nm), which causes tanning, UVB (medium wave, 280 to 315 nm), which causes sunburn, and UVC (short wave, germicidal, 100 to 280 nm), which is filtered out by the atmosphere and does not reach us. Incidentally, the ozone (O_3) layer of the atmosphere absorbs 97–99% of the UV in the range 200 nm to 315 nm, which is why the destruction of the ozone layer by some chemicals is dangerous for life on earth.

Solar Radiation Spectrum

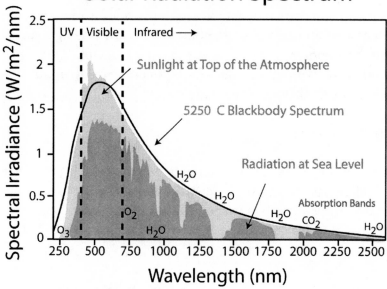

Not everything UV light does to you is bad

Ultraviolet light (between 270 nm and 300 nm) reaching our skin breaks down 7-dehydrocholesterol flowing in the bloodstream, converting it into vitamin D. Experts believe that our efforts to decrease skin damage by limiting sun exposure are pushing us into vitamin D deficiency. Sunscreen and dark skin interfere with our capacity to make vitamin D, but unless we work outdoors, we may not get enough sun even if we don't wear sunscreen. Talk to your doctor, and they may prescribe vitamin D or simply tell you to get a supplement. You will probably need 2,000-4,000 IU, so the 400 or 500 IU in your multi-vitamins may not be enough. But don't pass on sunscreen, because this is unlikely to solve your vitamin D problem (especially if you are dark skinned), and because skin cancer and skin aging are not nice.

It is known that lying in the sun can make you feel good. I'm sure that's why I see people lying in the sun for hours, even though they look red and puffy. It can't possibly be just to show their friends that they have money for a vacation in the sun, right? This *sunbathing addiction* may be related to the release of endorphins as UV reaches our skin. That fleeting sense of well-being is not worth the *elephant skin* and, worse, *melanoma*, which years of sunbathing may bring. For more in-depth information about UV damage, see Chapter 7, Skin pigmentation.

Oxidation and aging

When it comes to skin aging, there are two main culprits: UV light and oxidants, and much of the damage caused by UV light happens through reactive oxygen species (ROS*), chemically reactive molecules containing oxygen), so fending off ROS* is crucial to skin aging and health.

Whatever the owner of an oxygen bar may tell you, you and your skin have as much oxygen as you need. The concentration of oxygen in ambient air is 21%, and for anybody with healthy lungs and skin, this is more than enough. Prolonged exposure to oxygen partial pressures higher than normal will cause oxidative damage to lipids and cell membranes, eye damage and more. Our bodies have not evolved to contend with oxygen concentrations higher than what is already present in the atmosphere. Moreover, even current oxygen concentrations may cause oxidative damage, because when we use oxygen in respiration, the process is not perfect and ROS* are produced. We do have systems to cope with these oxidants, but these systems aren't perfect either.

What is oxidative stress?

ROS* are formed as a natural byproduct of respiration (breathing), and our body (including skin) has the means to deal with them. However, during times of environmental stress, like exposure to UV or heat, ROS* levels can increase dramatically, causing significant damage to cell structures. This syndrome is known as oxidative stress.

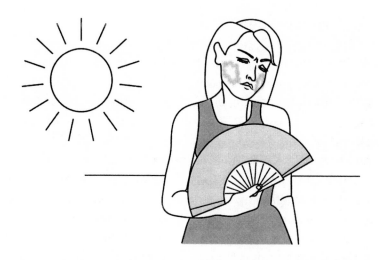

ROS* are also present in the atmosphere, especially in polluted environments and, incredibly, in some "skin care" products. Exogenous ROS*, those originating outside the body, are formed from pollutants, tobacco smoke, or ionizing radiation. Inside the body, the electron transport chain in the mitochondria is the major source of superoxide production in the cell. As electrons pass through the electron transport chain, a small fraction escape and prematurely react with molecular oxygen, resulting in the production of superoxide.

ROS* initiate destructive chain reactions

When a ROS*radical reacts with a fatty acid, the product of this reaction, reacts readily with molecular oxygen, creating a peroxyl-fatty acid radical, another ROS*. This new ROS* is also an unstable species that reacts with another free fatty acid, producing a different fatty acid radical and lipid peroxide, or a cyclic peroxide if it had reacted with itself. This cycle of ROS* reacting with other chemicals and forming more ROS* continues, as the new fatty acid radical reacts in the same way. What this means for us is more and more damage to structural lipids and membranes.

How bad is oxidative stress for your skin?

When ROS* production exceeds the cellular antioxidant capacity, in other words when there are more ROS* than your cells can handle, there will be oxidative damage to cellular components such as proteins, lipids, and DNA. DNA damage in particular, including single-strand lesions, deletions of bases, or "cross-links" between DNA and proteins. DNA damage is the basis of UV-induced skin carcinogenesis. Lipid peroxidation affects phospholipids both structurally and functionally and results in cell membranes with altered elasticity and permeability. Protein changes are reflected in the skin by a decrease in total amount of proteins, and alterations of the structure of proteins that are crucial to skin function (like collagen and elastin). Mitochondrial damage by ROS* leads to decreased energy production and even cell death.

Should you worry about oxidative stress? If you live in a polluted city, smoke, spend a lot of time in traffic, or if you go out in the sun without sunscreen - the answer is *yes*.

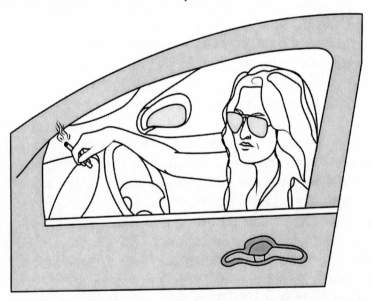

Antioxidants: the scavengers of ROS*

The formation of ROS* is prevented by an antioxidant system that includes **small antioxidant molecules** (ascorbic acid, glutathione, tocopherols), plus **enzymes** that regenerate the reduced forms of antioxidants, and disarm ROS* (superoxide dismutase or SOD, peroxidases and catalases). Antioxidants act as a cooperative network, employing a series of redox reactions. For example, in plants, there are interactions between ascorbic acid and glutathione, and between ascorbic acid and phenolic compounds.

Plant sourced antioxidants

We humans depend a lot on plants for antioxidant power, which we consume as food or apply topically. Plants have antioxidants because they need them for some of the same things humans do; they have an electron transport chain just like us for respiration, and photosynthesis has its own electron transport chain; this means ROS* everywhere! You will find lots of plant-made antioxidant chemicals in the list of Skin Actives ingredients, including polyphenols and terpenes with subcategories including flavonoids (EGCG, apigenin, quercetin), stilbenes (resveratrol), carotenoids (astaxanthin, lycopene and beta carotene) and more.

Astaxanthin gives our sea kelp coral its color. Astaxanthin is similar to some pigments that give coral exoskeletons their color. This is not just a similarity in color but also in chemistry. Most corals obtain the majority of their energy and nutrients from photosynthetic unicellular algae, called zooxanthellae, that live within the coral's tissue, and these algae also produce pigments that protect the coral from the sun. Because of its particular molecular structure, astaxanthin serves as an extremely powerful antioxidant. It has a very effective quenching effect against singlet oxygen, a powerful scavenging ability for lipid and free radicals, and effectively breaks peroxide chain reactions. Carotenoids are effective at low oxygen concentrations, complementing the activity of vitamin E which is effective at higher oxygen concentrations. Astaxanthin has also been shown to enhance and modulate the immune system. The antioxidant and immunomodulating activities, in combination or separately, may help reduce the acute inflammation reaction in the skin, and tissue just beneath the skin, that follows excessive exposure to UV radiation.

Skin problems related to ROS*

There are too many to enumerate, but they include wrinkles, sun spots (also called liver spots and age spots), vitiligo (loss of skin color in blotches), gray hair, and more. Any type of cell is susceptible to damage to its DNA leading to changes in the proteins, be it enzymes or structural enzymes, and damage to the system of cell membranes will affect cell function in general.

How much oxygen do we want?

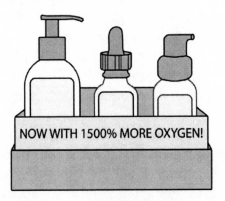

NOW WITH 1500% MORE OXYGEN!

We want to preserve a status in which ROS* are *allowed* to fulfill their job as defenders against infection and as intracellular second messengers, without overwhelming the natural antioxidant systems and leading us into oxidative stress. The last thing we want is to overwhelm our anti-oxidant resources with topical hydrogen peroxide or benzoyl peroxide. When your skin absorbs peroxides, the number of fibroblasts will decrease, and this particular cell that is essential for cleaning and repairing damaged tissue. In short, peroxides are an out-of-date tool whose time has passed.

What's so special about Skin Actives? The enzymatic scavengers of ROS*

Most skin care products include antioxidants, usually vitamin E or ascorbic acid or one of many botanical antioxidants. In addition to many more small molecules with antioxidant activity, Skin Actives offers purified, high specific activity superoxide dismutase, catalase, glutaredoxin and methionine sulfoxide reductase.

Why enzymes? Isn't astaxanthin good enough? Enzymes are proteins that can accelerate the rate of specific chemical reactions that would otherwise go too slowly to be compatible with life. In the laboratory, reactions can be accelerated by changing temperature or acidity of the medium, but life has strict constraints, which in humans means about 98 degrees Fahrenheit and pH around 7.0. Skin Actives Scientific offers a comprehensive list of enzymatic antioxidants that complement our body's own antioxidant system. A schematic description of how these enzymes interact with each other, with ROS* and with small molecules like glutathione, is depicted in the following figure.

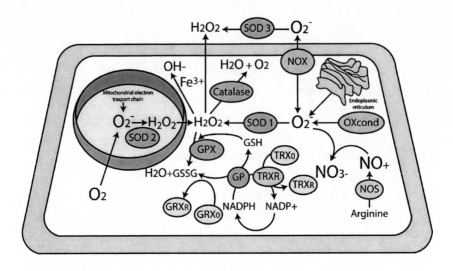

Enzymatic scavengers of reactive oxygen species (ROS*) with their cellular localization: cytosolic, mitochondrial and extracellular. Nitric oxide (NO·) has functions that overlap with ROS*, is synthesized from L-arginine and oxygen by enzymes called NO synthases and is one of the reactive nitrogen species (RNS*)

Superoxide dismutase - in our cells, we have our own SODs, but we can protect our skin by supplementing them with topically applied SOD. The size of the SOD used in skin care varies between 10,000 and 30,000 molecular weight, which is relatively small for an enzyme but large enough to be excluded from live cells. The fact that SOD is unlikely to enter live cells is not a problem. Lipid peroxidation occurs everywhere in the skin, not just in the live cells. The role of SOD is to eliminate the free radicals resulting from lipid peroxidation and to prevent the chain reactions that would eventually reach deeply into the skin, and topical application of SOD will certainly help to achieve this aim.

Thioredoxin.– Thioredoxins are proteins that act as antioxidants by facilitating the reduction of other proteins by cysteine thiol-disulfide exchange. Thioredoxins are found in nearly all known organisms and are essential for life in mammals. This is an enzyme I became familiar with in my days as a plant biochemist, long before

Wikipedia (or the internet, for that matter) was invented. Thioredoxin is "everywhere," including the regulation of the most abundant protein on earth, rubisco (the enzyme that "fixes" carbon dioxide, making life possible for every plant and animal, including us). Thioredoxin will make sure that the chain of events keeping proteins in their "right" reduction state is kept well oiled. Or, in other words, thioredoxin will facilitate the reduction of your skin proteins by cysteine (in a disulfide bond|thiol-disulfide exchange). The Trx (thioredoxin) and Grx (glutaredoxin) systems control cellular redox potential, keeping a reducing thiol-rich intracellular state, which no generation of reactive oxygen species signals through thiol redox control mechanisms.

Glutaredoxins (GRX) are small redox enzymes of approximately one hundred amino-acid residues which use glutathione as a cofactor. Glutaredoxins are oxidized by substrates and reduced non-enzymatically by glutathione. In contrast to thioredoxins, which are reduced by Thioredoxin reductase, no oxidoreductase exists that specifically reduces glutaredoxins. Instead, glutaredoxins are reduced by the oxidation of glutathione and reduced glutathione is then regenerated by glutathione reductase. Together these components form the glutathione system. Glutaredoxins function as electron carriers in the glutathione-dependent synthesis of deoxyribonucleotides by the enzyme ribonucleotide reductase. Moreover, glutaredoxins act in antioxidant defense by reducing dehydroascorbate, peroxiredoxins, and methione sulfoxide reductase (also supplied by Skin Actives). Beside their function in antioxidant defense, bacterial and plant GRX were shown to bind iron-sulfur clusters and to deliver the cluster to enzymes on demand.

L-Glutathione (gamma-L-Glutamyl-L-cysteinyl-glycine) is a tripeptide composed of the amino acids L-glutamine, L-cysteine, and glycine. Glutathione is part of the antioxidant defense system of the cell, together with superoxide dismutase, catalase, alpha-D-tocopherol (vitamin E), ascorbic acid (vitamin C), and others. Glutathione is crucial to cell life, and impairment of the glutathione system results in damage to the cell membrane and cell death.

The use of purified proteins is uncommon in the industry, because pure proteins can be very expensive. Because of the expertise of scientists at Skin Actives, we can synthesize and purify these proteins and make them available to our clients at a very reasonable price. As you will see later, we also use our expertise to synthesize and purify other valuable proteins used in skin care: human growth factors.

The most remarkable antioxidant ingredient, unique to SAS: The ROS* Terminator

The ROS* Terminator works to destroy ROS*, the potent oxidants that can harm our skin in many different ways. The key ingredients in our ROS* terminator are: sea kelp (lactobacillus/kelp ferment filtrate) bioferment, *Porphyridium* extract, fucoxanthin, astaxanthin, glutathione, plus purified thioredoxin, glutaredoxin, superoxide dismutase, and catalase.

Antioxidant Serum

We have now incorporated our ROS* Terminator into the Complete Hydrophylic Antioxidant Serum serum. The key ingredients are: magnesium ascorbyl phosphate (vitamin C), tetrahydrocurcuminoids, ferulic acid, epigallocatechin gallate (EGCG from green tea), hesperidin methyl chalcone, lycopene, glutathione, thioredoxin, glutaredoxin, superoxide dismutase (SOD), and catalase.

Antioxidant Day Cream

If we use a cream as a carrier, we can add to this cream an even better antioxidant mix, including both hydrophilic and lipophylic antioxidants, plus our very best botanical antioxidants. The key ingredients are: soy isoflavones, alpha lipoic acid [R(+)], ubiquinone (coenzyme Q10), resveratrol, pterostilbene, tocotrienols, alpha-D-tocopherol (vitamin E), astaxanthin, lycopene, lutein, beta carotene, *Centella asiatica* extract, superoxide dismutase (SOD), catalase, and glutathione.

Add individual antioxidants to your own formulation

Search the keyword *antioxidant* on our website for actives that will enrich your DIY product, making it better than anything you can find in a department store. Starting with ascorbic acid and derivatives (our favorite: magnesium ascorbyl phosphate), açai extract, R-alpha lipoic acid, amla extract, apigenin, and so much more.

Chapter 7: Skin pigmentation

Myth: Sunblock/sunscreen completely protects your skin
Can any sunblock truly protect you from the sun and prevent damage from UV light? **Absolutely not.** Sunscreen (a more suitable term than sunblock) helps protect the skin from the sun, lengthening the time it takes for the sun to burn and inflame the skin. But, sunscreen or no, if you spend time in the sun *uncovered*, your skin will pay the price.

Another myth: get a tan and you will be OK to go into the sun

Tanned skin will protect you from the sun so that you can spend hours sunbathing. No. At best, a suntan can provide the equivalent of a sunscreen with an SPF of 2 to 4. No complete protection from the sun exists.

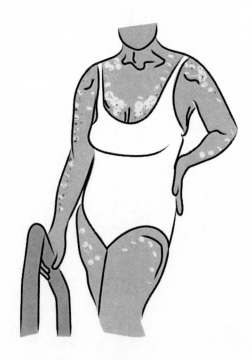

Skin pigmentation, a brief overview

The color of our skin is partly due to the pigment called melanin; other factors are the content of carotenoids in the diet, the bluish-white color of connective tissue, the abundance of blood vessels in the dermis and the color of blood flowing in them (which comes from oxy- and deoxy-hemoglobin). Other minor pigments (minor unless you have a bruise) present are bilirubin, the yellow degradation product of hemoglobin that colors bruises; the complete sequence includes hemoglobin to biliverdin to bilirubin to hemosiderin.

The different skin colors among individuals and races do not reflect major variation in numbers or size of melanocytes, but rather different kinds and amounts of melanin produced by the melanocytes. There are about 150 genes involved in the regulation of skin color in mice, including transcription factors, membrane proteins, enzymes, and several kinds of receptors and their ligands, and it is likely that these genes are still relevant in humans. This complexity, plus the troubled relationship of humans with skin color explains the many inconsistencies I have seen in the scientific (and not so scientific) literature on the issue.

Evolution favored the accumulation of more and darker melanin in the skin of humans living near the equator, where UV radiation is much higher than nearer the poles. Brown or black skin protects against high levels of exposure to the sun, while sun exposure more commonly results in melanomas (tumor of melanin-forming cells, typically a malignant tumor associated with skin cancer) in lighter-skinned people. The protective aspect of melanin is also at play when it comes to eyes. Melanin in the iris and choroid of the eyes helps protect from UV and high energy visible light; people with light colored eyes are at higher risk for sun-related eye problems, like cataracts.

Melanin is a good response to UV, and it is inducible by it via the response we call *tanning*. In old Europe, tanned skin was a sign of lower class, because people working in the fields were tanned and the owners of the fields were not. Conversely, in the 1950's tanning became fashionable, so the tan was still a class indicator but in the opposite direction. I hope that tanning will go out of fashion for good as the effects of too much UV exposure on skin are so damaging.

In many cultures and countries, lighter skin is still an indicator of class, and because of this, *skin lightening* is a billion dollar industry. In fact, many people risk their health for the *promise* of lighter skin; there are plenty of examples of dangerous chemicals and finished products used for skin lightening.
On the other hand, skin brightening is also important to people who develop uneven pigmentation, like melasma (the appearance of discolored patches on the face, typically triggered by hormonal changes during pregnancy and by sun exposure), pushing them to try risky remedies. For example, chemical peels and laser may cause further hyperpigmentation in people with darker skin. This is why we think it's important that we have healthy and safe ways to control pigmentation.

What does skin pigment do?

The color of our skin has been for millennia a major factor in inter-human relationships (and fodder for racists), but the pigments have an actual physiological role: protection from UV light. Melanin absorbs UV across a wide spectrum with the highest absorption in the shorter wavelengths that are most associated with DNA damage from UV.

UV light reaches human skin and leads to inflammation, DNA mutations and more. Reactive oxygen species (ROS*) are induced in the skin by solar UVA and UVB radiation and have long been suspected of contributing to the deleterious effects of skin damage by sunlight. ROS* promote lipid peroxidation, protein oxidation (with changes in structure), enzyme inactivation and DNA damage. For example, singlet oxygen mediates the UVA induction of inflammatory cytokines which in turn increase collagenase (a protease that breaks down collagen) in the skin. These effects of ROS* result in decreased cell viability and biological function, increased degradation of the dermal extracellular matrix, skin carcinogenesis and aging.

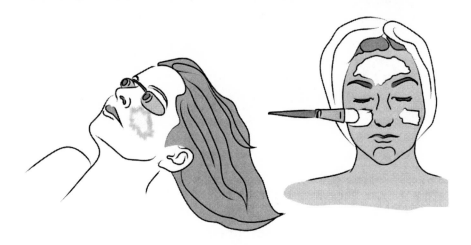

People take health risks by always trying to achieve what they don't have - tanning is detrimental to skin (UV radiation causes cellular damage) and those who use "bleaching" chemicals like hydroquinone risk developing a permanent condition where skin darkens and becomes resistant to lightening.

Does dark skin require special care?

Yes. And more caution when choosing skin care products.
A large percentage of skin problems are related to inflammation and inflammation can happen to any skin, whatever its color. Acne is a skin condition that involves inflammation, and when acne heals it is often followed by hyperpigmentation.

UV damage is accompanied by inflammation, and as the inflammation subsides it will often be followed by hyperpigmentation, with size and intensity varying. Melasma, the appearance of discolored patches on the face typically triggered by hormonal changes during pregnancy, use of anticonceptive pills and by sun exposure, seems to be more of a problem in Latino women.

For hyperpigmentation, the effects may be more noticeable in dark skin, but the worst effect of UV damage, melanoma, is more frequent in people with light skin.

Main causes of uneven pigmentation:

Aging

With skin aging comes dark spots (commonly referred to as sun spots, age spots, or liver spots) but also areas with loss of pigmentation, because mutations caused by UV in some areas lead to excess melanin production and accumulation, but in other areas melanocytes may have been lost or damaged. These changes are often irreversible, but some deep peels are followed by a healing process in which undamaged stem cells (present inside the pores) replace the damaged skin. SAS trichloroacetic acid peel can do this for you if you treat a small area. For larger areas you will need an MD.

Melasma

Genetics, visible light, UV, hormonal changes, and/or laser treatment can all contribute to this condition. The hormonal influence, via pregnancy or by birth control pills may be weaker than previously thought. Melasma is often inherited and even visible light appears to affect it; apparently there is more than just melanin involved, as vascularity increases in areas of melasma. It is interesting that tranexamic acid, a medication used to control blood coagulation, seems to help with melasma. Unfortunately, long term use of this drug is dangerous as is often the case with drugs that affect several aspects of human metabolism simultaneously.

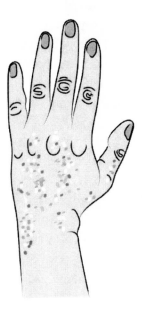

Sun damage

UV light reaches human skin and leads to inflammation, DNA mutations, and more. Reactive oxygen species (ROS*) are induced in the skin by solar UVA and UVB radiation and have long been suspected of contributing to the deleterious effects of skin damage by sunlight. ROS* promote lipid peroxidation, protein oxidation and protein cross-linking, enzyme inactivation and DNA damage. For example, singlet oxygen mediates the UVA induction of inflammatory cytokines which in turn increase collagenase (an enzyme that breaks down collagen) in the skin. These effects of ROS* result in decreased cell viability and biological function, increased degradation of the dermal extracellular matrix, skin carcinogenesis and aging.

If you are over 50 and had beach vacations, look at the sun-exposed side of your arm: patches of hyperpigmentation, whitish areas where there is little melanin, and wrinkles, plus a little scar made by your dermatologist when they excised a dark, menacing looking mole. Now look at the *shaded* side of your arm and you will find mostly youthful, elastic and smooth skin.

Ultraviolet light stimulates melanin production and the melanin formed absorbs the UV radiation in sunlight, so it somewhat protects the cells from further UV damage. However, significant melanin production takes about a week, so during the first day on the beach your skin is fully exposed to the fiery sun, and unprotected by melanin. After that, the suntan may give you the equivalent of an SPF of 2 to 4.

Sunburn is a delayed erythema (red skin) caused by UV B, which induces an increase in blood flow beginning about 4 hours following exposure. The underlying cause of this vascular reaction is damage to the cell from photochemical reactions and the generation of ROS*. There is damage to DNA, and several inflammatory pathways are activated, particularly those involving prostaglandins, leading eventually to vasodilatation and edema. Sunburn is not only painful, it is also a marker for severe UV damage and a predictor of worse things to come (like skin cancer) within years or decades. Why? There is a correlation between erythema and DNA damage; the UV wavelengths more efficient at producing erythema are also the most effective at forming pyrimidine dimers, which are followed by mutation. There is a link between a history of repeated, severe sunburn and increased risk for melanoma and non-melanoma skin cancer, and you can find out more about sun spots (aka solar lentigos) in Chapter 12 (Good news: You *can* turn back the clock).

Post-inflammatory pigmentation

Acne sufferers are familiar with this problem, in which acne lesions are followed by reddish to brown pigmentation areas. Some "home remedies" tried by melasma sufferers may also cause hyperpigmentation, because heating, laser applications and peels all lead to stress and inflammation. One of the mediators for this process may be endothelin 1 (ET-1), a peptide produced by keratinocytes after exposure to inflammatory factors or UV exposure that stimulates melanogenesis.

Vitiligo

This is a condition that causes loss of pigmentation of sections of skin. It occurs when melanocytes die or are unable to function properly. Vitiligo is not a well understood condition and a confirmed cause is unknown, but autoimmune mechanisms, oxidative stress and viruses may be contributing factors. At present, there is not a good treatment for it. Please visit the dermatologist; they will be up-to-date as new treatments arise. Please remember that once melanocytes die it is very hard, if not impossible, to recover pigmentation, and if you were to limit your medical care to *natural remedies*, you could miss out on useful treatments that a dermatologist may be able to offer.

Antioxidants may help in some circumstances and for this particular skin problem, we suggest our carefully crafted antioxidant products: Olive Anti-Inflammatory Cream, Antioxidant Day Cream and Antioxidant Serum, our most powerful antioxidant product. Try these products, but get permission from the dermatologist first. Also, you must avoid stress to your skin, especially from stressors like UV light, benzoyl peroxide and strong anti-acne products, which lead to the formation of free radicals. It is worth trying our Olive Anti-Inflammatory Cream, because inflammation is somehow involved in vitiligo. And try our Antioxidant Cream and Antioxidant Serum, because free radicals may be responsible for the disabled melanocytes. Always use our products for at least 2 months before giving up; it takes time to change the physiology of the melanocytes and for new skin to show. It may take even longer for *dormant* melanocytes to start producing melanin.

There has been a long-lasting controversy over whether melanocytes in vitiligo are actually lost, or still present but functionally inactive. Recent research using immunohistochemical techniques on skin biopsies suggests that about half the cells in the epidermis of vitiligo patients contain melanocytes in the affected area, and there are also melanocyte precursors (stem cells) present. In that case, the objective is getting the melanocytes to function properly, not easy, but the prospects are better than they would be if melanocytes were absent rather than malfunctioning.

Reference:

Seleit, Iman; Bakry, Ola Ahmed; Abdou, Asmaa Gaber; Dawoud, NM (2014) Immunohistochemical Study of Melanocyte-Melanocyte Stem Cell lineage in Vitiligo; A Clue to Interfollicular Melanocyte Stem Cell Reservoir. Ultrastructural Pathology, 38: 186-198.

Dark under eye circles

The causes of dark under eye pigmentation vary widely, but research suggests that the following types are most common. The vascular type is characterized by the presence of redness in the lower eyelids with prominent capillaries or bluish discoloration due to visible blue veins. In the constitutional form there is brown-black hyperpigmentation of the lower eyelid skin along the orbital rim. Post-inflammatory hyperpigmentation is usually caused by allergic contact dermatitis. Shadow effects can occur due to the shape of the face or a deep tear trough. There is also skin laxity, dry skin, hormonal disturbances, nutritional deficiencies and chronic illnesses all of which can affect coloration and appearance of the eye area.

The skin of the eyelids is the thinnest skin in the body, and that makes it special. Whatever happens in that area will show more than anywhere else in the face. Our eyes are a focal point in our face, we even look at this area with more attention that we pay to the rest of the face.

Blood vessels can be seen through the thin skin. Inflammation will affect this area more. If a blood vessel leaks even a bit, the hemoglobin in the blood cells will be transformed into pigments that will stay beneath the skin for a long time, and these pigments can be seen through the thin skin, a part of the "dark under-eye circles" that may make us look tired and even sick.

With age, the skin gets thinner and the very thin skin of the eyelids will become even thinner, and will show our age more than the rest of the face.

So, do you need a special skin care for the eye area? I think so. One that will preserve the dermal matrix, with hyaluronic acid and collagen peptides. There are actives that will help maintain the elasticity and integrity of the blood vessels, like horse chestnut's escin, grape seed proanthocyanidins and hesperidin methyl chalcone. Rosehip oil will provide some essential fatty acids. Chrysin will help dissolve pigments derived from hemoglobin. Liquid crystal will give your skin radiance while also providing essential molecules to the cell membranes. And lots of anti-oxidants to fight the free radicals produced by our own body or those that surround us in the busy city. Also, this area is more sensitive than the rest of the face, so alpha lipoic acid, a great active that can "sting", has to be used at very low concentration in the eye area.

What can you expect from Skin Actives' Bright-I Cream? Some of the actives also present in other Skin Actives products to promote skin nutrition, (sea kelp bioferment, hyaluronic acid, natural active peptides), and synthesis and protection of skin proteins and structural polysaccharides. Other actives promote cell replication, like epidermal growth factor and retinyl acetate because the thinner skin of the area is also why capillaries are more visible, contributing to the appearance of dark under-eye circles. Others actives have general antioxidant properties but also display specific properties that make them especially useful for the delicate eye area.

Actives in Skin Actives Bright-I Cream: sea kelp bioferment, caffeine, retinyl acetate, hesperidin methyl chalcone, natural active peptides, grape seed proanthocyanidins, sodium hyaluronate, chrysin, epidermal growth factor (EGF), antioxidant booster, liquid crystal, glutathione, Pal-GQPR (palmitoyl tetrapeptide), retinyl acetate, a retinoid and a form of vitamin A, will accelerate skin renewal, preventing the formation of milia and "erasing" wrinkles. Caffeine is a great active: it promotes efflux of sodium, promotes fat mobilization, has analgesic properties, antioxidant activity and more. One of my favorite aspects of caffeine is that it promotes post-replication repair of DNA, one reason why caffeine helps prevent cancer. Chrysin activates the enzyme uridine diphosphate-glucuronosyltransferase (UGT1A1) that leads to the degradation of bilirubin, a product of the breakdown of blood hemoglobin that may have been released by broken capillaries. It also suppresses histamine release, and "puffy" eyes are a very common complaint. Lecithin is in this formulation to provide the lipids your skin needs. Lecithin taken orally seems to help decrease serum cholesterol, but it does not work when injected into lipomas (a benign tumor made of adipose tissue), and it will not make fatty thighs go thin. However, some Skin Actives clients say it works well on fat deposits under the eyes. Remember that topical application of caffeine can decrease the thickness of subcutaneous fat, so even if lecithin does not work for you, our Bright-I Cream may. If you are desperate (it is always a bad idea to feel desperate when making any decision, even buying skin care), try SAS Cellulite Control Cream. Hesperidin methyl chalcone is an effective antioxidant that decreases capillary fragility and permeability. This does not mean that you should feel free to rub your eyes when you are sleepy, rubbing eyes is a "no-no". Glutathione, a great natural antioxidant that fulfills crucial roles in our body, is always helpful, especially in polluted environments like a big city or the highway.

If you have dark under-eye circles caused by broken capillaries, using Bright-I Cream will improve them or clear them completely (the same properties will help erase bruising, because the actives will help clear the tell-tales signs of blood leaks). If your dark circles are hereditary and caused by melanin pigmentation, our Bright-I Cream will not help you much, but you could try our Skin Brightening Cream.

For general skin laxity (a problem that can take you to a plastic surgery in search of a blepharoplasty) go for Vitamin A Cream and Collagen Serum. And remember, rubbing your eyes when you are sleepy is a bad idea.

How to prevent uneven pigmentation

Prevent skin damage of any kind (burns hot or cold), avoid inflammation, prevent damage by UV: wear sunscreen. Be physically gentle to your skin, avoid scarring, don't "overclean". Prevent and treat acne with our Salicylic Wash, Acne Control Cream, Acne Control Mask, T-Zone Serum, and Zit Ender. Don't let acne continue; treat it with powerful products that don't have side effects. Get your recommended 8 hours of sleep (always a good idea).

What to do after the fact

Many dermatologists will go straight to the triad of hydroquinone, retinoids and corticosteroids. We at SAS insist on safety, we do like retinoids and we have created a Vitamin A Cream that is non-irritating. For anti-inflammatory activity we don't use corticosteroids, and for skin brightening we don't use hydroquinone. We have, however, formulated a UV Repair Cream that will help heal skin following hours (and years) of damage. By keeping up with the scientific research we can introduce promising new skin lightening ingredients that are also *safe*, like soy protease inhibitor, salicin, glutathione, carotenoids, baicalein and more.

What NOT to do

Skin lighteners, skin whiteners, and skin brighteners are different names given to a type of product that decreases skin pigmentation.

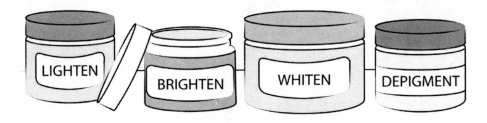

There are two kinds of people looking for skin lighteners, those with irregular pigmentation resulting from age spots and/or melasma, and those who are not content with the color of their skin. There are several mechanisms by which a substance can help to lighten the skin color, but most of them work by suppressing melanin synthesis. Some chemicals are very effective but can be irritating or are known to have undesirable side effects. For example, strong chemicals may end up bleaching the skin permanently and irregularly, or increasing pigmentation in spots. The best way to avoid bad results is to not use strong chemicals like hydroquinone, especially in types of skin known to react badly, like African American and dark Latino skin.

What we want from our ingredients is specificity, and effects restricted to the area of application. One big problem with treatment of skin hyperpigmentation is that consumers are always looking for fast, easy, miraculous solutions. You will not get this with skin lighteners of uncertain origin. Illegal and restricted substances are often present in cosmetics sold for skin bleaching, like hydroquinone, tretinoin and corticosteroids. Those who buy imported cosmetics for strong skin whitening are exposing themselves to products contaminated with clobetasol propionate and hydroquinone and may suffer from their negative side effects.

SAS Skin Brightening Cream addresses multiple factors

Skin pigmentation is a very complex process that involves different types of cells and the transport of chemicals between them. Because of this complexity, there are multiple ways to affect the overall process and the mechanisms of action of the actives used to decrease pigmentation are also complex. The following is an attempt to convey that complexity.

We added ingredients to the Skin Brightening Cream that act as antioxidants. In general, antioxidants decrease pigmentation by preventing the oxidative polymerization of melanin intermediates. Antioxidants can also regulate the signaling process by scavenging ROS* in the skin. Tocopherol and other lipophilic antioxidants prevent lipid peroxidation in cellular membranes and increase the intracellular glutathione content. Our ROS* terminator containing glutathione exerts its action as a skin whitening agent at various levels of melanogenesis which include interference with cellular transport of tyrosinase, inactivation of the tyrosinase by binding with the copper-containing active site of the enzyme, and mediating the switch mechanism from eumelanin to phaeomelanin production. Magnesium ascorbyl phosphate lightens melasma and solar lentigos and has been shown to have a protective effect against skin damage induced by UV-B irradiation. Mangiferin is a xanthone, a potent antioxidant. Alpha lipoic acid, has been reported to prevent UV-induced oxidative damage, mainly through the down modulation of NF-kB activation. In addition it inhibits tyrosinase activity possibly by chelating copper ions.

We have also included ingredients that compete with the substrate for tyrosinase. Arbutin decreases tyrosinase activity by acting as an alternative, unproductive substrate for tyrosinase. Kojic acid dipalmitate releases kojic acid in the skin and also acts as an inactive, alternative substrate for tyrosinase. Glucosamine inhibits the glycosylation required by tyrosinase to be active. Unsaturated fatty acids like linolenic acid inhibit melanogenesis through increased tyrosinase degradation by the proteasome.

Chemicals with anti-inflammatory activity like salicin inhibit both COX-1 and COX 2 and is a representative non-steroidal anti-inflammatory drug used to treat pain. It has also been shown to inhibit tyrosinase expression and enhance tyrosinase degradation. Brown algae contain sulfated polysaccharides that can regulate plasma levels of endolethin-1. Baicalein is a flavonoid extracted from the root of skullcap, a key herb in Chinese medicine (huang qin), and it inhibits ET-1 production and ROS* formation. Bisabolol inhibits UVB-induced pigmentation by inhibiting ET-1 effects. Luteolin is a flavonoid contained in various kinds of plants, it inhibits the gene expression of ET-1. Melatonin has been shown to inhibit processes driven by cyclic AMP in pigment cells and has anti-inflammatory properties.

The final group of ingredients is responsible for the inhibition of melanosome transfer: niacinamide (vitamin B3) and active soy extract.

Because melanin synthesis increases as a response to stress of several kinds, like UV and oxidants, it is a good idea to avoid the sun and use sunblock. In the case of melasma, it seems that visible light (not only UV) may have some influence, so it is best to use a physical sunscreen - one containing zinc oxide. You should also remember that skin brighteners do not destroy existing melanin, so you will have to wait until your skin renews itself to be able to see the lighter skin.

Pigmentation modifiers to avoid

TGF-beta-1

Melanosomes are specialized organelles in which melanin is synthesized and deposited. The addition of TGF-β1 to cultured melanocytes produced less pigmented melanosomes even when the cells were concomitantly treated with αMSH to increase their fully melanized melanosomes. However, TGF-beta 1 is not a good candidate for skin lightening because of its multiple effects on the whole cell. TGF-beta 1 is a multifunctional peptide that controls proliferation, differentiation, and other functions in many cell types. TGF-β1 plays an important role in controlling the immune system, and has different effects on different types of cells and even on cells at different developmental stages. Pigmentation modifiers that also affect other cell processes are not useful in the treatment of pigmentation disorders.

Topical corticosteroids

Topical corticosteroids have strong anti-inflammatory effects. They have been used for the treatment of melasma to decrease irritation caused by hypo-pigmenting agents and work by suppressing cytokines through the inhibition of nuclear factor kappa B (NF-κB) activation. Topical steroids can be effective by the suppression of cytokines such as endothelin-1 and GM-CSF, which mediate UV-induced pigmentation. Unfortunately, they can only be used short term, because of the numerous side effects.

Tranexamic acid

Tranexamic acid (trans-4-aminomethyl cyclohexane carboxylic acid) is a plasmin inhibitor, commonly used as a haemostatic agent owing to its antifibrolytic action and is also promoted as a systemic skin whitening agent especially as oral or intradermal injections for melasma. It is a synthetic derivative of lysine. Plasmin is a protease that enhances the intracellular release of arachidonic acid, a precursor of prostanoid, and also elevates alpha-melanocyte stimulating hormone (α-MSH) processed from proopiomelanocortin. Both arachidonic acid and α-MSH can activate melanin synthesis by melanocytes. Tranexamic acid by way of its antiplasmin activity depletes the keratinocyte pool of arachidonic acid involved in ultraviolet (UV) induced melanogenesis. It is not safe to use it for a long duration in view of its anti-hemorrhagic property resulting in side effects like venous thromboembolism, myocardial infarction, cerebrovascular accidents and pulmonary embolism.

Another major question is whether switching, long-term, the normal machinery from eumelanin (which is protective against UV radiation) to pheomelanin (it has been suggested that this form favors UV-induced DNA damage) by an external agent like tranexamic acid, could result in an increased incidence of skin cancers.

Hydroquinone

Hydroquinone has been used for decades as a skin lightening agent, but mid-term effects (i.e. in a matter of months) are worrying: in about 70% of the users, there is deposition of yellow-brown pigment in the dermis, in addition to break-down of collagen and elastin. The chemical composition of the very dark material in ochronosis and the mechanism by which hydroquinone promotes its formation are unknown. Hydroquinone may also cause skin and renal cancer.

Chapter 8: Let us do no harm

Primum est ut non nocere: in medicine and surgery "let us do no harm."
- Quote attributed to Thomas Sydenham (1624-1689) by Thomas Inman in Foundation for a New Theory and Practice of Medicine, 1860.

Every medical and pharmacological decision carries the potential for harm. This applies to the skin, an organ in the human body. We may think modern medicine is a continuation of the medicine of antiquity, but it isn't. Up to the 1860's, medicine was a game of mirrors that in practice accelerated the death of the patients who had money to pay for "medical" care. The set of treatments was limited to bloodletting, purges, emetics, mercury and little else. In fact, poor people were in a better situation: they had no choice but to allow nature to take its course, and they usually fared better.

What changed in the 1860's? Some primitive statistics were finally allowed into medicine, so that doctors could see that their actions were killing patients. After a lot of resistance, doctors allowed science to influence medical practice: anesthesia and vaccines were introduced, germ theory led to changes in the treatment of infectious disease, and in 1930 antibiotics were introduced in medical treatment (see "Bad medicine: doctors doing harm since Hippocrates", by David Wotton, 2006, Oxford University Press). Only then did medicine truly start helping people, alleviating pain, delaying death, and improving quality of life.

Skin care: OK to do harm?

Taking into account that modern medicine is relatively new, it is not surprising that old practices still survive here and there. But when it comes to skin care, I see old practices everywhere, often causing harm. In skin care, scientific discoveries are often used as advertising tools rather than as information for improving skin health.

Skin care, very often, is "bad skin care". We at Skin Actives receive many alarming emails that have led me to believe that people often put common sense aside when it comes to skin care. Otherwise, why would a woman continue to "moisturize" her skin when it turns bright red and hurts every time she performs this "treatment"?

Despite long term research showing that benzoyl peroxide, a skin sensitizer, promotes tumor growth and causes breaks in the DNA strands, it is still used by many skin care companies. One of these companies tried to justify using strong oxidants by saying that "Phenyl radicals are not as damaging as hydroxyl radicals, and since the reaction leading to damage occurs quickly, the damage is brief and fleeting." Although expected, this is a ridiculous defense of their use of a harmful ingredient in a skin care product.

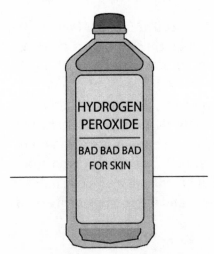

Conversely, we have many situations in which a beneficial ingredient is discarded because of silly reasons, such as being petroleum derived (nothing wrong with that) or replacing safe preservatives with extracts adulterated with unsafe preservatives. The industry seems capable of creating an infinite number of distractions, accusations and lies in their effort to conquer a little bit more of the market.

We have to accept that the skin care business is a human activity and, as such, it is not always honest. The public then needs to be better prepared to oppose such tactics and choose the right treatment. Examples of skin care treatments that can do more harm than good are peels, alcohol based toners, laser procedures, facial threading, benzoyl peroxide, micro-needling and more. Doesn't this list remind you of the other list: "bloodletting, purges, emetics, mercury"?

Looking for magical herbs

We look back at ancient medicines for information about plants that may be beneficial to our health. But please don't assume that old medicine is better than new: in ancient times, people used whatever was on hand to cope with illness and infections, this does not mean that what they were using was beneficial (although I am sure that placebos have always been helpful).

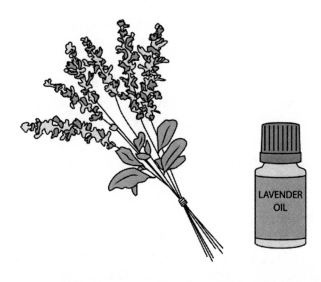

Lavender is commonly considered to be calming to our skin, but to a small percentage of the population it is an irritant that yields allergic reactions.

So, what about cosmetic companies that look for magic cures for aging skin in rare plants? Unless they know a lot about phytochemistry they may end up hurting you. I always hope that they use these plant materials only for their label value and that there is actually no significant amount of toxic chemicals in them.

It is somewhat fitting that a British skin care company (that shall not be named) uses magic to make magic. In their advertising for a product line they make with an adventurous title (let's call it Griffin's Blood) they promise "sculpting" of the face, as if our faces were mounds of butter in a county fair. But they can't do sculpting, look at the complex structure of our head and face and see what it would take to sculpt into bone, cartilage, fat, skin, and muscle.

But sure, let's use magic to do magic. How about *Griffon's Blood*? This is the common name of a red colored resin that has been used for centuries as a dye, varnish, and to make paint: *Croton lechleri* resin. This resin, a latex, can be used to seal wounds, because the latex dries quickly and acts as a bandage. If I were in the Amazon and got hurt, maybe I would use this "sangre " (blood). But this does not mean that I would use it on my face here in the city. *Croton* extract is a complex soup of chemicals with interesting activities, including antiviral and antiherpes; but long term use can cause problems, including DNA mutagenesis, the last thing we need in skin that has been damaged by the sun and is already full of mutations.

Some chemicals in *Croton* are cytotoxic (toxic to cells). Cytotoxic is not always bad, sometimes you want to kill cells, like in cancer. When trying to medicate a serious problem, like some life threatening complications of AIDS (one of the uses of this ingredient) it is worth taking a risk. But if your objective is to rejuvenate your skin, go for proven and safe actives: look at our collagen serum actives, for example, and don't apply cytotoxic agents to the skin which has already suffered innumerable mutations as a result of sun damage.

There are some nice antioxidants in this latex (flavanols), and maybe with time it will be possible to purify the beneficial chemicals. Only then may you see a resin in SAS products.

The price of skin care and the placebo effect

Historians said that when old medicine did good, it was through the placebo effect. The same is true of much skin care these days. One of our consultants responded to my query about an article in the New York Times regarding possible differences in effectiveness between brand name prescription vs. generic. The reply reminded me of a very well known effect in skin care: the *luxury factor*.

Here is the relevant portion of the reply: "There are major problems with this article. There's a placebo effect with any medication that could be up to 30% or even more of the effect. There may be a different placebo effect if the patient switches from the expensive brand name to the generic (it's been shown that if a patient is told a medication costs more, they find it works better on their pain than a cheap medication - even when it's the exact same pill given to all patients in the study)."

Greenwashing

I first saw the term *greenwashing* used by a cosmetic chemist, Perry Romanowsky, to describe the efforts from the industry to hide preservatives from consumers who think they are savvy.

"The first form of greenwashed formulating is where you create a standard product but give it a green, natural, granola-crunching name. The driving belief behind this type of formulating is that consumers do not look at ingredient lists and are more focused on the product name and design. This is a slightly cynical form of natural formulating, however, it was regularly practiced in the mid to late 1990's by cosmetic companies. The reason? It was effective... It's the least expensive way to *formulate* a natural cosmetic product."

As Mr. Romanowsky discusses, there have been *enhancements* to greenwashing. In my view, they are even more cynical than simply calling a product "Honest" or "Seventh Generation" (granola-crunching names). They involve the use of a loophole in the INCI nomenclature that allows manufacturers to hide ingredients used as part of processing the final ingredient. For example, grapefruit seeds have no preservative power by themselves. However, using a series of chemical reactions, the substances in them can be converted into new chemicals, or the chemicals may simply be added but not listed. There is no resemblance in the chemical structure of grapefruit seed to this "natural preservative," but this is what the loophole is about. For example, benzethonium chloride, triclosan, and methyl parabens have been found in grapefruit seed extracts sold as preservatives. Extracts free of these chemicals had no preservative power (antibacterial/ anti-mold activity). It makes sense that if there are no chemicals with preservative power, the ingredient will have no preservative power, because there is no magic to preservation.

Don't ask me to use *Leuconostoc*/radish root ferment filtrate!

Preservatives are *essential* to the health of the consumer; they prevent the growth of bacteria and mold on the products that you apply to your skin. But the pressure to hide the preservatives from the ingredient lists is very strong, with some people who don't know about bacteria and mold insisting that preservatives are not necessary. The answer of honest companies is to explain the need for preservatives and to remind the consumer that a piece of bread, even when kept in the fridge, will eventually be covered in mold and bacteria. Dishonest manufacturers, on the other hand, hide the preservatives in a variety of manners.

How can a Lactobacillus (or Leuconostoc) ferment be used as a preservative? Lactobacillus ferment is what I would call the yogurt you eat every day. Leave yogurt in the fridge long enough and another bacteria and mold will grow on it. How can such a ferment be used as a preservative, at a very low concentration, to extend the life of a skin care product? It can't. But it is possible to cheat. Yogurt is a fermentation product of milk made by the activity of Lactobacillus. Just as yogurt is made, the Lactobacillus bacterium can be added to a *soup* that contains a synthetic chemical, undecylenic acid, which has anti-fungal activity. The name will still be Lactobacillus/radish root ferment filtrate. I have nothing against the use of synthetic chemicals or undecylenic acid, but I think it is fraud to hide preservatives in a way that causes the consumer to believe he/she is buying a *natural* product.

I'm sure that many companies that use this "natural" preservative and call their finished product "natural" don't know that this is not natural. However, ignorance shouldn't be an excuse, and manufacturers of skin care products should know their ingredients! When you buy a product containing Leuconostoc/radish root ferment filtrate, you should know that you are buying a product that contains synthetic preservatives. I am sure many more preservatives using this nomenclature loophole will keep coming, at least until the consumers *wise up*. How about elderberry or Japanese honeysuckle as bases? The nicer the name, the more "granola crunch" the name will be, but the name does not make the preservative any more natural.

References:

von Woedtke T, Schlüter B, Pflegel P, Lindequist U, Jülich WD. (1999) Aspects of the antimicrobial efficacy of grapefruit seed extract and its relation to preservative substances contained. Pharmazie, 54:452-6.

Jing Li, Chaytor JL, Findlay B, McMullen LM, Smith, DC, Vederas JC (2015) Identification of Didecyldimethylammonium salts and salicylic acid as antimicrobial compounds in commercial fermented radish kimchi . J. Agric. Food Chem., 63:3053–3058

What were they thinking?

In the old days, hydrogen peroxide was used to disinfect wounds, but then it was found that this procedure slows healing and leads to scarring because it damages cells. Nowadays we use hydrogen peroxide and other strong oxidants to bleach wood pulp and to remove spots from carpets, but not to disinfect wounds. We know that hydrogen peroxide is a reactive oxygen species (ROS*) and carries an oxidizing power that can be destructive.

Why would someone pay $85 for "Natural Brand" Oxygen Gel or $65 for "(Woman's Name)" Oxygen cream"? Advertising for "(Woman's Name)" Oxygen cream states that it "will provide your skin with 1% active oxygen", but why should we want to *oxygenate* our skin?

"Natural Brand" Oxygen Gel ingredients: water, denatured alcohol, dimethicone, cyclopentasiloxane, betaine, methyl gluceth-10, glycerin, propanediol, hydrogen peroxide, coco-caprylate, allantoin, C12-20 acid PEG-8 ester, plankton extract, carbomer, triethanolamine, C13-14 isoparaffin, lauroyl lysine, polyacrylamide, lecithin, laureth-7, cetyl phosphate, urea, lactic acid, sodium lactate, serine, pentylene glycol, sorbitol, sodium chloride, disodium EDTA, tocopherol, phenoxyethanol, ethylparaben, methylparaben, fragrance, butylphenyl methylpropional, linalool, hexyl cinnamal, alpha-isomethyl ionone, citronellol, limonene.

"(<u>Woman's Name</u>)" Oxygen Cream ingredients: water, mineral oil, glycerin, stearyl alcohol, polysorbate 20, hydrogen peroxide.

In these two products, the source of oxygen is hydrogen peroxide, H_2O_2, a very strong oxidizer and highly reactive oxygen species. Because it is so reactive, most living organisms have enzymes, catalases and peroxidases, capable of destroying hydrogen peroxide as it appears. Apparently, the people at these companies don't know about catalase, because they're trying to sell you a product containing hydrogen peroxide. They seem to think that your skin will benefit from the blockage of skin capillaries by oxygen bubbles. It won't.

On the one hand we have "Natural Brand" and "(<u>Woman's Name</u>)" trying to oxygenate your skin. And on the other, Skin Actives Scientific, selling an antioxidant cream (and the individual components) whose function is to eliminate strong oxidants like hydrogen peroxide. Science is on our side.

Chapter 9: The science of skin and hair care

Myth: DNA from X and stem cells from Y will help your skin!

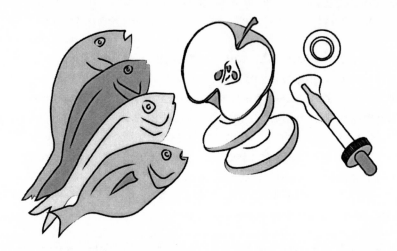

Any skin care product that includes DNA and stem cells is trying to take advantage of what is *in fashion*, but scientifically speaking - they're nonsense.

Your cells have your own DNA, which you inherited from your parents. Your cells will express certain genes, those that correspond to the organ, in this case skin, and time of your life (a baby doesn't express the same genes as an adult).

DNA that belongs to fish, cows or whatever, when applied to your skin, may be used by your skin but not to make fish proteins or cow proteins. Your immune system will not let anything reach the nuclei of your living cells; otherwise it would wreak havoc. Havoc is what happens when foreign DNA does actually get to the nuclei of your cells or when a virus cheats your immune system and manages to get in, but it isn't something that will happen when you apply a cosmetic to your skin.

What is it that the skin care companies are trying to sell to you? Extracts of apple stem cells or culture media (discarded after human stem cells were grown in it). Forget about those claims: our skin already has its own stem cells, and you will not benefit from anybody else's stem cells (one exception: people with some types of cancer affecting their immune system). Intact, not extract, plant stem cells will be very useful if you are thinking of growing some roots, or getting some leaves to take advantage of the beautiful sun out there. But make sure you are using stem cells (meristems) of the same species (a very similar variety may work). For example, a budwood with meristem cells from an existing tree could be grafted onto you, the rootstock. These meristems will allow you to grow shoots, flower and make lovely oranges for fresh juice every morning, *if you are an orange tree*. If you aren't an orange tree but a human, then I suggest you work at keeping your own stem cells as happy as they can be.

So what happens to the DNA that marketing persuaded you to apply to your skin? Most of it will be washed away; some of it will be broken down and your skin may absorb the components: nucleotides, sugars, phosphates, etc. The same thing will happen to the stem cells from a pear, cow, horse or whatever. If your immune system is working well, nothing will get in, unless it's broken down as food for your skin first.

This is one more example of how marketing uses a trend to promote useless ingredients. DNA and stem cells go directly to my "ARGHHHH" list. In a *CSI: NY* episode the murderer was discovered because she had received a stem cell facial (cow stem cells) before committing the murder. You can add this one to the list of reasons why you should *not* have a stem cell facial.

Stem cells

Stem cells are cells in multicellular organisms that can divide and differentiate into diverse specialized cell types. Stem cells can also divide to produce more stem cells. There are not that many stem cells in our adult bodies. Our epidermis basal layer contains stem cells; other tissues and organs that harbor small subpopulations (0.1 to 3%) of adult stem cells (progenitor cells) are vascular walls, heart, brain, skeletal muscles and adipose tissues as well as the epithelium of the eyes, lung, liver, digestive tract, etc.

What about our own, precious stem cells? They allow our skin to heal and renew. Unfortunately, they also age. Damaged by the environment, they can self-repair to a certain extent, and telomerase is not a problem. But UV exposure and stress of different kinds will affect stem cells, because they are not magic cells, they contain fragile DNA like any other cell. To keep your skin stem cells healthy, think about avoiding any further stress like sunbathing and make sure you use Skin Actives' UV Repair Cream.

Pores

What are pores? Why do we have them? Pore is the common name given to the pilosebaceous unit, a part of the anatomy of normal skin and different from the pores involved in sweating (which are much smaller and not often a cause of complaint). The pilosebaceous unit consists of hair, hair follicle, muscle, and sebaceous gland.

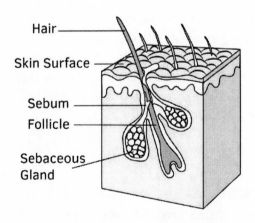

Sebaceous glands are connected to the hair follicle and deposit sebum on the hair, which brings the sebum to the skin surface along the hair shaft. In our less-evolved primate cousins, sebum protects and *waterproofs* hair and skin. For us, sebum still can help our skin with some anti-aging effects because our sebum waterproofs our skin, preventing moisture loss over time. Besides this benefit, sebum is mostly a leftover product of evolution, and how much we make and have is more up to genetics than it is to what we do to our skin. In any case, pores - and sebum - are here to stay for a few hundred thousand years, so we have to learn to live with them.

Why do we have larger pores than babies? Our pores get larger and more visible during adolescence, when sex hormones increase sebum secretion. Men and women produce androgens and estrogens, but starting before puberty the concentrations of sex hormones in the blood is different for boys and girls, and they will affect the skin metabolism through the receptors to which they bind with great specificity. As androgen production increases, sebum secretion increases too, pores get larger and comedones and acne come in. Men and women have both estrogens and androgens, so unless the receptors for androgens are missing (a relatively rare condition) most of us are likely to get comedones and acne, whether we are male or female.

Is there anything nice we can say about pores? Yes: they are the source of the multipotent stem cells responsible for maintaining skin structure throughout our life. When we hurt our skin in everyday life, these stem cells, abundant in the bulge region of the hair follicles (in the basal layer of the epidermis) will be activated and do the all-important repair and regeneration of the skin or start a new cycle of hair growth. Remember these important stem cells, they have your DNA and the genetic information required to repair your skin. Obviously, they cannot be replaced with apple stem cells or anything else, whatever the ads may say (unless you are an apple).

It's likely that the higher androgen level is responsible for the thicker skin that men have on practically all of the body, not just the face, and may be responsible for the fact that men's skin seems to age more slowly than the skin of women.

Another big factor is that estrogens, which affect the synthesis of hyaluronic acid and other dermis macromolecules, decrease sharply in women after menopause; while in men, the decline is slower.

The science of skin care: energy production in the cell

Mitochondria: sing. *mitochondrion*, from the Greek *mitos*, warp thread + Greek *khondrion*, diminutive of khondros, grain, granule.

In my opinion, mitochondria, antioxidants and protection from UV are the keys to keeping healthy skin healthy for the many years our skin has to do its job. In other words, the need to protect skin from UV and strong oxidants and to protect the integrity of mitochondria is NOT age specific. It's not practical to have several mitochondria creams to target different ages. It's easier to formulate the best possible mitochondria cream and *layer*, on top or below products to complement its action. For example, a woman of 50 may wish to layer Anti-Aging Cream on top of our Revitalizing Night Cream and also use our Collagen Serum and UV Repair Cream.

Let me explain why mitochondria are so important and so worth the best possible care we can afford. You may have read this information before because cell structure and energy production are so important to our lives, and to Skin Actives.

Mitochondria provide the energy as adenosine triphosphate (ATP), the form of energy our cells can use to do *housekeeping,* and also to grow and divide. This is true not just for us humans, but for all eukaryotes (organisms with nuclei). Mitochondria use molecular oxygen to extract a lot of energy that would otherwise be lost, and foodstuff is eventually converted to low energy water and carbon dioxide.

The science behind these statements is so complex and so awesome that you would have to study carefully several textbooks or read the Nobel lectures of many awardees to comprehend it. I am not trying to make it easy, that's impossible, but just to convey its importance.

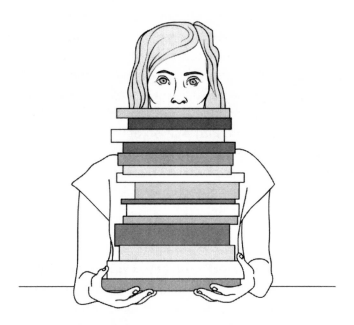

This great energy-converting efficiency comes at a cost: mitochondria produce strong oxidants like hydrogen peroxide and the superoxide and hydroxyl radicals as by-products. All of the cell's sophisticated antioxidant mechanisms (including vitamin C, glutathione and vitamin E and various antioxidant enzymes) can't completely protect mitochondria from slow but persistent damage. This oxidative stress makes mitochondria age at a faster pace than the rest of the cell, because oxidation of lipids, proteins, RNA, and DNA is faster. Indeed, oxidative damage to mitochondrial DNA (the only organelle with its own DNA outside the nucleus) is 8 to 10-fold higher than the damage found in nuclear DNA. Oxidative damage also affects adversely the inner mitochondrial membrane, where the crucial enzyme ATPase is located and where ATP is produced. The phospholipids of the inner mitochondrial membrane change and become even more sensitive to oxidative damage. These changes are bound to affect membrane fluidity and permeability and will certainly impair the ability of mitochondria to meet cellular energy demands.

Oxidant-induced acceleration of senescence has major consequences for mitochondria. Aged mitochondria lose efficiency at extracting the last bit of energy from foodstuff. Enzyme activity and substrate binding affinity decrease. It has been found that this decay in function can be partially reversed in aged animals by feeding them the mitochondrial metabolites acetyl carnitine and alpha lipoic acid, and information of this sort provides circumstantial evidence for the mitochondrial theory of aging (a.k.a. free radical theory of aging) which states that the slow accumulation of impaired mitochondria is the driving force of the aging process.

Even if we don't accept the theory that mitochondrial aging is the cause of overall aging, there is no doubt that deterioration of mitochondria is at least responsible for the aging of the whole organism. Up to now, this information has been translated into the topical application of alpha lipoic acid, acetyl carnitine and various antioxidants in anti-aging skin care products. We at SAS take the effect of oxidants on the cell very seriously: we have been offering acetyl carnitine and alpha lipoic acid both as pure chemicals and in ready-to-use skin care products. We also broadened the spectrum of antioxidants (see for example Antioxidant Booster) and lipids (ELS Serum) for the prevention and reversal of skin damage. The addition of mitochondrial concentrate to our actives and ready mixed products is a natural step in the efforts of Skin Actives Scientific to bring the benefits of scientific knowledge and technology to our clients. The cream's orange / yellow color comes from the mitochondria and from coenzyme Q10. It feels silky and absorbs extremely well.

Why sirtuins are important for your skin

Sirtuins are proteins with a very sophisticated role in the cell: they control the enzyme that converts acetate, a source of calories, into acetyl CoA, a key point of entry to cellular respiration. See what Wikipedia has to say about these proteins:

"Sirtuins may be able to control age-related disorders in various organisms and in humans. These disorders include the aging process, obesity, metabolic syndrome, type II diabetes mellitus and Parkinson's disease. Development of new agents that would specifically block the nicotinamide-binding site could provide an avenue to develop newer agents to treat degenerative diseases such as diabetes, atherosclerosis and gout."

For the time being, I am not planning on testing the most effective anti-sirtuin strategy so far: calorie restriction. Apparently, near starvation extends life.

The potential role of sirtuins in aging made them an instant hit with the skin care industry. Even when research on sirtuin-related pharmaceuticals is still in its infancy, there is a "pro-sirtuin technology" included in a famous brand. Obviously, there is no real pro-sirtuin technology in there, as none exists, but the product contains a couple of interesting actives, i.e. *Andrographis* extract and resveratrol. Ignore the usual marketing gimmicks and go for *Andrographis* and resveratrol because they are good, at SAS we use these two ingredients also. *Andrographis* is an excellent active, which I appreciate very much for its anti-allergic activity.

There are two main actives to consider in relation to sirtuins: niacinamide and resveratrol.

Again, from Wikipedia:

"Normally, sirtuin activity is inhibited by nicotinamide, a component of vitamin B3 (also known as niacin), by binding to a specific receptor site. Drugs that interfere with this binding should increase sirtuin activity. It is known that resveratrol found in red wine, can inhibit this interaction and is a putative agent for slowing down the aging process. However, the amount of resveratrol found naturally in red wine is too low to activate sirtuin, so potential therapeutic use would mandate purification and development of a therapeutic agent".

Two comments on this paragraph:

1) There is more to niacinamide than its effect on sirtuins, and niacinamide is too good to eliminate from our skin's diet, so you must look for other ways to stimulate sirtuins without eliminating niacinamide.

2) Skin Actives Scientific already sells purified resveratrol.

Your lips

Why do you need anything for your lips? Aren't your lips just like the rest of your skin? Not really. The skin of the lips, with their three to five cellular layers, is very thin compared to typical face skin, which has up to 16 layers.

The lip skin does not have sweat glands or hair, so it does not have the usual protective layer of sweat and body oils which keep the skin smooth and somewhat protected. For these reasons, the lips dry out faster and become chapped more easily.

And why the color? In people with light skin color, the lip skin contains fewer melanocytes (cells which produce melanin which give skin its color). The blood vessels can be seen through the skin of the lips, which makes them look pink/red, and the resistance to UV provided by the melanin will not be there to protect them.

Your lips are exposed to stress of different sorts: sun, smoke, hot liquids. Stress makes them more susceptible to infections like herpes virus. SAS provides you some tools to protect your lips. What will you gain? You can prevent and even reverse to some extent the effects of sun, aging and tobacco consumption, i.e. lip lines and inflammation.

All about hair

Hair matters greatly to how we see ourselves and how others see us. Hair is produced by live cells in our scalp, but by the time the hair sees the outside world, there are no live cells in it. Most of the actives provided by Skin Actives or anybody else can't do much for it except for providing some extra protection. Still, *just* protecting your hair is worth the trouble because if you wear it long it may have to last for years from the time it is formed until you cut it or it falls naturally.

Hair growth begins inside the hair follicle, and the only *living* portion of the hair is found in the follicle. The base of the root is called the bulb, which contains the cells that produce the hair shaft. The hair follicle includes the oil producing sebaceous gland which lubricates the hair and the muscles responsible for causing hairs to stand up in goose bumps.

Hair follows a specific growth cycle with three phases: anagen (active), catagen (transition), and telogen (resting) phases. Each phase has specific characteristics that determine the possible length of the hair. All three phases occur simultaneously. In our scalp, one strand of hair may be in the anagen (active) phase, while another is in the telogen (resting) phase. During anagen, the cells in the root of the hair are dividing rapidly, adding to the hair shaft. The anagen phase lasts between 2 and 7 years (for some individuals even longer), waist-length hair or longer is only possible to reach for people with long anagen.

The hair that is visible is the hair shaft, which shows no biochemical activity and for this reason is considered *dead*. The cells formed in the hair bulb are now mostly keratin. As hair keratin is synthesized, it assembles into rope-like intermediate filaments. The structure of these filaments provides strength to the hair shaft. As determined by their amino acid sequence, the protein molecules twist to form a very stable, left-handed superhelical (a coil that coils itself into another coil) motif that assembles with other such units forming filaments consisting of multiple copies of the keratin monomer. In addition to intra- and intermolecular hydrogen bonds, keratins have large amounts of the sulfur-containing amino acid cysteine, required for the disulfide bridges that confer additional strength and rigidity by linking into permanent, thermally-stable super-structures.

As you can see from this summary description, keratin structure (not completely elucidated to date) makes hair so resilient that it can resist harsh conditions like those encountered in daily life. Hair will grow for years without noticeable damage, although UV light will bleach the melanin in the hair shaft and lighten hair after a sunny summer.

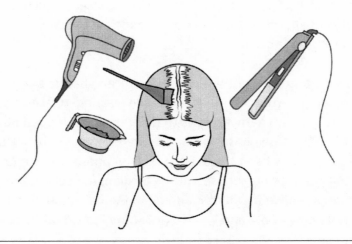

As soon as humans started grooming their hair, *culture* demanded that we expose hair to heat (!), bleach and dyes (!!), strong chemicals (!!!) and traction (!!!!). That's right: these are not natural stresses but the result of treatments dictated by fashion. Still, there's no reason why these harsh treatments should affect the capacity of your scalp to produce new, healthy hair, unless the chemicals, heat, etc. reach the scalp and damage the cells capable of producing hair. Just try to be sensible and remember that your scalp and hair have to last for many, many decades.

Conditioners contain chemicals with positive electrical charges that will cling to the hair. The chemicals in the conditioner collect on the edges of the damaged scales of the cuticle, helping to smooth over and fill in the breaks and cracks. As a result the hair tends to become more manageable and shiny; proteins and dimethicone are useful in this process. Colored or permed hair needs extra care, and conditioners and other products can help by *patching up* the damaged hair cuticle.

Panthenol is absorbed into the hair and helps retain moisture and antioxidants will protect the hair from oxidants in the environment, although no antioxidant is a match for the strong oxidants used to modify hair color and shape. It is possible to change the shape of the hair (in a perm or hair relaxer) by denaturing keratin, using chemicals to break down the disulfide bridges that give keratin its strength, and letting the disulfide bridges re-form after the hair is given a new shape. Since perms were invented, milder and less noxious chemicals have been created to break down the keratin structure and reform it in the desired shape. Strong chemicals are also used to color hair, increasing the permeability of the hair so that it can absorb the dyes; the process involves the use of strong oxidizing agents (peroxides) and alkali.

Try to avoid unnecessary damage to the capacity of your scalp to keep forming new hair. Take measures to prevent the strong chemicals used in perms and coloring to come into contact with the scalp. Whatever you do, don't try to *save* money on a perm or hair color, it can cost you dearly.

Shampoo is needed to clean your hair, but first, do no harm: shampoos shouldn't contain strong detergents like sodium dodecyl sulfate that can damage the scalp by extracting structural lipids.

The science of gray hair

Following the discovery that follicles lacking in two crucial antioxidant enzymes make gray-white hair, we added these two enzymes to our Hair Care Serum that should help protect your scalp and prevent the loss of hair color.

To respond to clients' questions: we will not be making any effort to patent this extraordinary serum, because the Patent Office will reject applications that are derived by using common sense on published scientific discoveries, and our serum is a clear example of common sense. However, you should not expect this type of product to be forthcoming from other skin care or hair care companies because, besides common sense, the two key actives in this serum present a major achievement that is not easy or cheap to replicate outside of SAS.

Gray hair happens because there is little or no melanin incorporated in the hair as it is being formed in the follicle. It has been known for some time that oxidants were implicated in the damage and death of the melanocytes in the follicle, and new evidence shows that hydrogen peroxide (H_2O_2) accumulates in the hair shafts of gray-white hair. Two enzymes are involved in the prevention and repair of oxidative damage: catalase and methionine sulfoxide reductase. In gray hairs, these two enzymes are almost completely gone.

Catalase breaks down hydrogen peroxide, preventing damage to the cell's DNA and membrane lipids. On the other hand, methionine sulfoxide reductase (MSR) repairs protein damage. For example, MSR can fix a damaged amino acid in tyrosinase the key enzyme of melanogenesis. Another way of preventing damage of tyrosinase by hydrogen peroxide is to have L-methionine in the environment.

Reference:

Wood, J. M., Decker, H., Hartmann, H., Chavan, B., Rokos, H., Spencer, J. D., Hasse, S.,Thornton, M. J., Shalbaf, M., Paus, R., Schallreuter, K. U. (2009) Senile hair graying: H_2O_2-mediated oxidative stress affects human hair color by blunting methionine sulfoxide repair. FASEB Journal 2009 Jul; 23:2065-75. doi: 10.1096/fj.08-125435. Epub 2009 Feb 23.

Keratinocyte growth factor

This growth factor has been proven to stimulate hair growth in laboratory studies. It also accelerates healing and increases skin volume. It may also help prevent hair loss during radiation therapy during cancer treatment. Keratinocyte Growth Factor (KGF) binds to the KGF receptor on the cell surface. It acts as both a growth and survival factor by stimulating epithelial cell proliferation, differentiation, and migration and promoting a number of cell protective mechanisms.

KGF is also known as FGF-7 and heparin-binding growth factor-7. KGF is a member of the fibroblast growth factor family and has been found to stimulate hair growth. Cells that respond to KGF do so because they have receptors on the cell membrane that recognize the growth factor, normally produced by cells near or far from the target cell. The binding of the growth factor to the receptor initiates a cascade of molecular events that will eventually lead, among other effects, to cell division. Keratinocyte growth factor has been shown to regulate proliferation and differentiation

in epithelial tissues and may regulate the stem cells of the hair follicle.
References:

Braun, Susanne, Krampert, Monika, Bodo, Enikoe, Kuemin, Angelika, Born-Berclaz, Christiane, Paus, Ralf, Werner, Sabine. (2006) Keratinocyte growth factor protects epidermis and hair follicles from cell death induced by UV irradiation, chemotherapeutic or cytotoxic agents J Cell Science, 119: 4841-4849

Danilenko, Dimitry M.; Ring, Brian D.; Yanagihara, Donna; Benson, William; Wiemann, Bernadette; Starnes, Charles O.; Pierce, Glenn F. (1995) Keratinocyte growth factor is an important endogenous mediator of hair follicle growth , development, and differentiation. Normalization of the nu/nu follicular differentiation defect and amelioration of chemotherapy-induced alopecia. American Journal of Pathology 147: 145-54

SAS products for hair care

Sea Kelp Coral, in a serum, conditioner or by itself will help with itchy scalp. Your scalp is where everything begins: healthy hair follicles will make healthy hair. If your hair follicles are already damaged, take advantage of SAS actives and pre-mixed products.

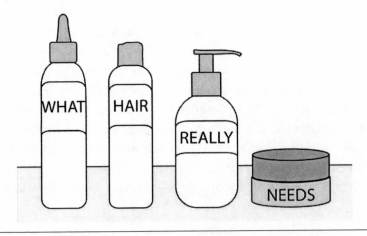

Our Hair Care Serum contains keratinocyte growth factor (KGF) in a medium that contains everything your hair follicles need: vitamins, amino acids and much more. KGF, also known as FGF-7 and heparin-binding growth factor-7 (HBGF-7) and a member of the fibroblast growth factor family, completes the serum. KGF has been found to stimulate hair growth. Chrysin and grape seed proanthocyanidins help with poor scalp micro-circulation, follicle atrophy caused by dihydrotestosterone, and follicle aging. Nutrients are included in the serum to compensate for the decline in blood irrigation to the scalp as we age. Most cancer fighting therapies interfere with fast cell division and they will affect hair, so if a friend or family member that will undergo this type of treatment, ask her/him to discuss with the doctor using this serum, the KGF in the serum will help retain hair during and after radiation treatment.

Our serum for gray hair contains antioxidant enzymes in a medium formulated to decrease the oxidative stress to your hair follicles and the cells that make the hair. SAS Gray Hair Serum contains catalase, methionine sulfoxide reductase, phloretin, L-methionine and other actives. The objective of our Gray Hair Serum is to prevent the loss of hair color. There is no evidence that anything can restore the original color to gray hair, but there is room for hope. If the color loss is relatively recent, the non-oxidant environment provided by our serum may prevent the death of melanocytes and allow tyrosinase in those melanocytes to do its job again.

It used to be that we only discussed bacteria when speaking about infections. In skin care, it was all about acne and how to kill *Propionibacterium acnes*. Now, you can see bacteria and the "microbiome" everywhere in magazines to advertise skin care products.

Human skin functions as a physical barricade to stop the entry of pathogens, but also hosts innumerable commensal organisms (commensal means living in a relationship in which one organism derives food or other benefits from another organism without hurting or helping it). The skin cells and the immune system constantly interact with microbes maintaining an equilibrium, despite a continuous change in the environment.

Skin bacteria

Bacteria are essential to the function of the human body, and many species live in us, and on us. We are familiar with the negative effect of taking oral antibiotics on our gastrointestinal tract and the flora that resides there. The probiotic supplement market is booming and even major yogurt brands now carry probiotic formulas.

The type of bacteria depends on the part of the body and on the person, but there will be many in each part, living in peace with each other and with us. Many factors influence the composition of the microbiome, like diet, gender, the environment including ultraviolet radiation, family and other factors that will impact the species composition.

In the skin, many bacterial species will not grow well in culture, so a complete identification of bacteria requires the use of DNA technology. The dry skin surface is dominated by *Proteobacteria, Actinobacteria, Bacteriodetes*, and *Firmicutes*. Moist areas are rich in *Staphylococcus* and *Corynebacterium* spp. A lower bacterial diversity is seen in oilier sites, suggesting that only few bacterial communities, like *Propionibacterium*, can flourish under those conditions; in acne the problem is the abnormal proliferation of this bacterium.

Scientists are getting to know more about the skin microbiome but it will be a lot of research and a long time before we know enough to effect a positive change.

Also, just in case you are not doing it already, stop using antibacterial soaps. Frequent use of some antibacterials will promote the development of bacteria resistant to antibiotics, promoting the proliferation of drug resistant infections, a scourge of medicine.

Chapter 10: Skin problems

The aim of this chapter is to help you understand how the skin works and what happens when it "malfunctions". Nothing in this chapter can replace your MD. Please see your MD if you have concerns.

Eczema and atopic dermatitis

We need our immune system to defend us from the infectious agents that are trying to invade us, like bacteria, viruses or fungi. Sometimes the immune system does not work as well as we would like it to, and it plays tricks on us.

The terms eczema, atopic dermatitis or atopic eczema are used to describe a chronic inflammatory skin disease with allergic causes, in which the skin itches and there is some scaling, crusting and/or oozing (rather than just erythema or inflammation). Skin affected by eczema is more prone to bacterial infection, as the skin barrier breaks, facilitating attack by microorganisms.

People who have eczema also tend to have other manifestations of allergy, like allergic rhinitis or asthma. Atopic dermatitis is very frequent, affecting about 10% of the population, and it can start as early as 2 months of age.

Atopy is characterized by high concentrations of serum immunoglobulin E (IgE), a high incidence of IgE-mediated responses on skin testing to common inhaled antigens and many other manifestations of an oversensitive and "skewed" immune system. For the time being, there is little that can be done about atopy at the molecular level, but if things get tough we can always go for one or more of the over the counter medicines available.

What can you do if you or a loved one has atopic dermatitis? It may help to avoid common allergens such as dust mites, animal danders and saliva, mold and pollen. Children can have food allergies so it is worthwhile to explore this aspect with the help of an MD, always remembering that "exclusion diets" can deprive the child of essential nutrients. Immunotherapy, i.e. desensitization with "allergy shots", does not seem to work for atopic dermatitis, in contrast to its relative success in treating patients with other allergic disorders.

Avoid factors that may worsen atopic dermatitis: excessive bathing, low humidity environments, emotional stress, dry skin, rapid temperature changes, and exposure to solvents and detergents. Doctors do not agree on whether showering or bathing is preferable in patients with atopic dermatitis. Some doctors recommend a hydrating bath followed by immediate application of emollients, and others recommend a shower of short duration, which better removes surface antigens that may be acting as trigger factors.

The itchiness of eczema leads to scratching, and scratching leads to rashes. This vicious circle must be stopped because the scratching can lead to permanent changes in the skin, including scars, and infections. Although cortisone is a good idea for emergencies, it cannot be used long term because it may lead to skin thinning, depigmentation, and stretch marks. Also, corticosteroids will reach the bloodstream, suppressing the activity of the adrenal glands.

Evaporation of skin humidity leads to dry skin in patients with atopic dermatitis, and this is why skin hydration is a key component of overall management. Lotions have a high water and low oil content and can worsen dry skin via evaporation, thus triggering flares of eczema. Conversely, thick creams with low water content, or ointments, which have zero water content, protect the skin better against dryness (and eczema flares). Apply emollients immediately after bathing to keep the skin well hydrated.

To alleviate the itching you can use Skin Actives Scientific Sea Kelp Coral, calamine, rosehip or pomegranate seed oil, or take a warm bath with Beta Glucan (from Oat) and Rosehip Seed Oil. To decrease inflammation, use Anti-Inflammatory Cream. There are many actives that seem to help with eczema, have a look in our glossary.

Acne

Just because a skin condition is *common*, that doesn't mean that it isn't *serious*. What happens to one's skin happens in front of the world, and acne is a good example. Acne affects a large proportion of the population, but again, just because something is common, that doesn't mean it isn't serious. Serious acne can ruin a teenager's life.

Though acne is a normal skin condition, what's significant about it is that it makes us so unhappy. And while advertising promises miraculous results, the companies that produce the ads clearly stand to benefit by painting pretty pictures to catch desperate people. There are no miracles to be found in the real world. There is no easy solution, or cure, for acne. The good news is that we know enough about acne to *control* it, and this is a great achievement.

In order to maintain a leading edge in the skin care industry I constantly evaluate products and ingredients that are marketed as *new* and *innovative*. I have three main sources of information regarding ingredients. The ingredient lists for thousands of products on the market (while reading thousands of ingredient lists is boring, it's also reassuring because it shows that we're still the best). I also consult scientific publications that report on how chemicals, synthetic or natural, affect processes related to acne. Our own clients and forum members who write to me suggesting new actives are my final source. Nobiletin was brought to my attention in this way.

The skin care industry continues to introduce *new* products, but whatever the name of the new products that will perform *miracles* on your skin, it always comes back to salicylic acid and/or benzoyl peroxide. So the old saying is fitting: nothing new under the sun. Usually, there is a *stinging* ingredient (menthol or a derivative) added to make you think that *something* is happening. These stinging ingredients can only make things worse, because stinging has no beneficial effect on the acne lesion and at high concentration they can increase inflammation.

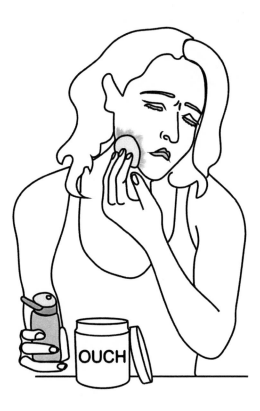

If there is a danger in the usual anti-acne products – it's that *fast buck* companies don't care about the long-term health of their clients' skin. They will use benzoyl peroxide even if repeated use of a product with this ingredient will *aggravate* acne and age the skin prematurely. Benzoyl peroxide decimates the natural bacterial flora of the skin and ages skin by flushing it with a strong oxidant that will promote DNA mutations and other issues.

This is why you will find in our acne control kit the following actives: Oleuropein, wild yam and niacinamide have anti-inflammatory properties. Salicylic acid, salicin, and retinyl acetate normalize keratinization. Nobiletin, *Coleus* oil, galangal and granulysin decrease acne bacteria. Nobiletin, zinc and EGCG decrease sebum secretion. Yeast beta glucan is an immune response enhancer, making your skin more able to battle the acne bacterium. Saw palmetto, zinc and EGCG act as inhibitors of 5 alpha-reductase activity.

Don't look for the *miracle* active among them. They work well together - but no miracles, just biochemistry.

Pores and acne

One of the effects of this not-very-useful sebum is acne, so I can see why the popularity of pores is so low.

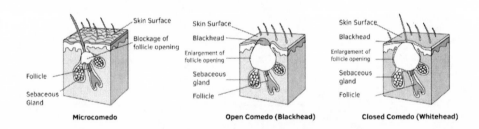

Microcomedo   Open Comedo (Blackhead)   Closed Comedo (Whitehead)

Pores get larger and more visible during adolescence, when hormones increase sebum secretion. Pores can get clogged with sebum, keratin, and dead cells, resulting in an environment lacking in oxygen and favorable to the growth of the acne bacterium, *Propionibacterium acnes*. The products of bacterial metabolism cause the inflamed pimples characteristic of acne. This is a real problem and one that adequate skin care can prevent and correct.

A comedo may be closed by skin - *whitehead* - or open to the air - *blackhead*. Being open to the air causes oxidization, which turns the lipids at the top of the "plug" black or brown.

How to "minimize" pores

If your skin is very oily, decreasing sebum secretion will decrease pore size in younger skin. Try our T-Zone Serum and see whether it works for you.

SAS Collagen Serum, used in conjunction with our Vitamin A Cream (or our Acne Control Cream, which also contains Vitamin A) will help with acne scars, including red marks and hyperpigmentation. This great duo will also help diminish the size of pores by decreasing sebum secretion and promoting synthesis of structural skin components that will build up at the edge of the pore.

As long as you continue using the Vitamin A Cream, you will not need strong exfoliators because Vitamin A will keep your skin cells renewing and the Collagen Serum will provide nutrition to make the skin renewal possible. Though your pores will never be again the size they were before adolescence, and your skin can never be again as smooth as a baby's, this pair of products, will help to *normalize* the shedding of external layers.

If you live in a polluted city, our Cleansing Oil will remove makeup and clean skin, pores included. Our Vitamin A Cream will exfoliate slowly; you will not see the exfoliation - as it is chemical instead of physical, but it will happen. Pores will be unclogged, healthy and free of infection.

Makeup and Photoshop can help maintain the *illusion* of *no-pores*. Some inert ingredients help reflect light in such a way that pores are hidden. There is no reason why this type of makeup should cause any problems.

Avoid products containing alcohol like many toners. They may promise to *shrink* your pores, but the way they do so is by dehydrating the skin. Alcohol will also dissolve and remove valuable lipids from your skin, and in the long term it will dry the skin and then sebum secretion may increase.

Rosacea

This is a chronic skin disorder that affects more than ten million Americans, with almost half of the sufferers aged between 30 and 50 years old. The disease has been called "the Celtic curse" because it affects people of Northern European descent more often. Women are more likely to suffer rosacea of the milder form, and men more frequently have the severe form, which involves deformity of the nose. Rosacea nearly always appears on sun damaged skin.

Except for cases precipitated by use of steroids, the causes of rosacea are not known, but there are several discredited theories, including those involving skin mites (*Demodex folliculorum* and *Demodex brevis*) and the bacterium *Helicobacter pylori*. Because we do not know what causes the disease, there are no good treatments, and all that can be done is to prevent irritation and inflammation.

Rosacea develops in stages and is characterized by "twitchy" blood vessels, i.e. subcutaneous blood vessels that are too sensitive. Almost anything will start flushing and blushing episodes, followed by redness of the skin caused by congestion of the capillaries and chronic dilation of capillaries causing elevated dark red blotches on the skin. Rosacea patients may develop severe sebaceous gland growth that is accompanied by papules, pustules, cysts, and nodules. Inflammatory lesions develop in the areas of erythema and may look like acne, but in rosacea there are no comedones, the primary event in acne.

It can be difficult to distinguish acne, eczema, and other skin afflictions from rosacea. It is however, very important to recognize rosacea because, although it cannot be cured right now, early recognition and treatment can prevent progression to disfigurement.

There are several medical treatments used to attenuate the effects of rosacea rather than cure it. Azelaic acid is effective in the treatment of rosacea, particularly at the stage when there are papules and pustules. Laser treatment may help with telangiectasia and deformation of the nose.

What can you do about rosacea? It is important to avoid precipitating factors such as exposure to sun, stress (easier said than done!), cold weather, hot beverages, cigarette smoke, alcohol consumption, and any foods that you have noticed exacerbate your rosacea. Any cosmetics used must be non-comedogenic and nonirritating. Use sunblock and avoid sun exposure, because sun damage is one of the factors that precipitate rosacea. Protect your skin from infection and weakening of the skin barrier as well.

Steroids are not an option, so to control inflammation try our Olive Anti-Inflammatory Cream or our anti-inflammatory actives, like Niacinamide. Try soothing actives, like Licorice Extract, or Green Tea Extract with Caffeine, which would work as a vasoconstrictor. *Centella asiatica* and Horse Chestnut extracts are well known for their capillary strengthening properties. Many clients have found relief using 4-ethoxybenzaldehyde mixed with a base cream. Azeloyl Glycine and Magnesium Ascorbyl Phosphate are other options. You could also try our Glycan-7 Booster, which may help with strengthening the skin barrier and enhancing the immune response against Demodex. Our clients have also reported excellent results with Sea Kelp Coral used on its own (please see our forum). Our Redness Reduction Serum with Epidermal Growth Factor works for others.

I usually ask clients to try these products one by one and see whether one of them helps. With such a complicated condition as rosacea, we should expect that at different stages the skin will respond in different ways to the same treatment.

Scars and the complicated process of wound healing

The quality of healing will depend on the communication between the cells and enzymes involved in the process of healing a wound. In the case of a visible scar, the process did not go the way we would have hoped. After a cut in the skin, there are four major stages of healing: clot formation, inflammation, proliferation, and maturation.

Healing of a wound starts with formation of a clot to stop bleeding and to reduce the likelihood of infection. Neutrophils, a type of white blood cells, invade the area within a day after the wound occurs, and cell division begins in epithelial cells after a day or so.

During the inflammatory phase, macrophages (also white blood cells) kill bacteria, remove damaged tissue and release chemicals, including growth factors that encourage fibroblasts and other cells to migrate to the area and divide.

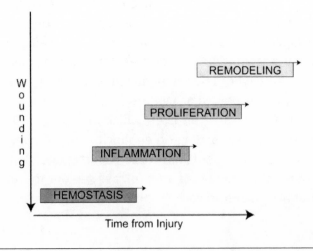

In the proliferative phase, immature granulation tissue containing plump active fibroblasts is formed from the edge of the injury and towards the center. The fibroblasts make abundant type III collagen, filling the defect left by the open wound.

As granulation tissue matures, the fibroblasts produce less collagen and become more spindly in appearance. They begin to produce the much stronger type I collagen. Some of the fibroblasts mature into myofibroblasts which contain the protein actin, allowing them to contract and reduce the size of the wound. Scar maturation can last a year or even longer. Unnecessary vessels formed for healing are removed by apoptosis (programmed cell death), and type III collagen is largely replaced by type I. Collagen, which was originally disorganized is cross-linked and aligned along tension lines. Ultimately, a scar made of collagen, containing a small number of fibroblasts, is left.

In acne scars, there is no cut, just inflammation. The inflammation damages the tissue that is fighting the bacterial infection. After the acne lesion heals, it can leave a red or hyperpigmented mark on the skin. The redness, or hyperpigmentation, is seen as the skin goes through its healing and remodeling process which takes approximately a year. If no more acne lesions develop in that area, the skin may heal normally.

After inflammation is over, bacteria, red blood cells and damaged tissue are removed by macrophages (a crucial step because if damaged cells or bacteria are left over more inflammation will be triggered). Blood vessels are repaired, and new cells form in the damaged site similar to the cells that had been damaged and removed.

There are several things you can do if a cut or minor surgery happen. Use the SAS Restoration Cream you keep in the fridge. The wound will heal much faster and be less likely to end as a visible scar as the epidermal growth factor and other actives make up for the delay in the healing process that comes with age.

For optimum wound care, the key requirements are to provide hydration, control inflammation, reduce tension and accelerate collagen synthesis. Micro-porous tape is used to replace sutures on wounds to reduce tension. This type of tape also allows for a healing gel or cream to be applied on the tape. Talk to your doctor about using SAS Restoration Cream at this stage. Show your doctor the ingredient list. After about a month, you may begin using our Scar Vanishing Gel.

A scar may look to our eyes like a finished event, but it isn't - the skin is live tissue. We can still intervene by inducing the synthesis of new collagen and the destruction of the old proteins. Retinoids in SAS Retinyl Acetate, Vitamin A Cream, and Vitamin A Serum can help and Collagen Serum and Scar Vanishing Gel may help reprogram your old scars and improve their structure and appearance.

For faster results (but requiring a relatively long recovery period of a week to a month), producing a new wound in the location of the scar may be the way forward. This is what a trichloroacetic (TCA) peel does. For small areas, try our TCA Spot Peel Kit. For larger areas, make sure you get an experienced and recommended practitioner, preferably an MD, to do the work. This may be the solution for a back scarred by acne during adolescence. But remember that TCA will wound your skin; you don't want this delicate work to be done by a helpful but inexperienced friend who will not know what to do if something goes wrong. And make sure you have SAS Restoration Cream on hand as the actives in it are an essential part of good healing.

Remember that skin is alive. Drastic procedures like dermabrasion or laser are available, but you must consider the possibility that any procedure could *cause* further scarring.

What are your expectations for a skin care product? It's good to consider this in advance, because if you're clear about what to expect, you're less likely to be disappointed.

Make-up refers to a product designed to hide skin imperfections. Depending on what you need to hide, the texture, thickness, and color will vary. Here, effectiveness means *cover*. To hide a scar, you need a thick product, while to hide a wrinkle, products with reflecting pigments may be enough. These products are also useful for temporary coverage of tattoos.

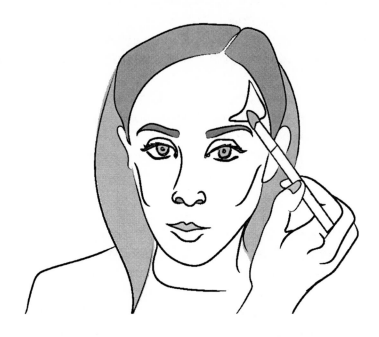

Look at the label of the product. Don't focus on the name, as names are chosen by marketing people to entice you to buy a product and usually have no connection to what the product can actually do.

Look at the ingredient list. Here are some sample ingredient lists:

Scar cream: dimethicone 2%, water, cetearyl alcohol, glycerin, C12-15 alkyl benzoate, dicaprylyl carbonate, pentylene glycol, cyclomethicone, arachidyl alcohol, alcohol, behenyl alcohol, arachidyl glucoside, onion extract, copper tripeptide-1, aloe leaf, cetearyl glucoside, tocopherol acetate, hydroxyethyl acrylate/ sodium acryloyl diethyl aurate copolymer, hydroxyethylcellulose, hydrolyzed soy protein, glycine, panthenol, hydrolyzed collagen, PEG-400, arginine HCL, leucine, lysine hydrochloride, alanine, sodium lactate, aspartic acid, glucose, glutamic acid, isopropyl alcohol, mannitol, sorbitol, tromethamine, valine, histidine hydrochloride, isoleucine, phenylalanine, tyrosine, potassium sorbate, sodium benzoate, citric acid, sodium hydroxide, fragrance.

This is a silicone-based cream that should work for *hiding* scars. Every ingredient after hydroxyethylcellulose, a thickener, is a "label value" ingredient to make you think that the product will *fix* you, or it is a preservative or a fragrance. There are also thicker products that contain pigments that match the skin color, to help with more pronounced or colored scars.

Another list: water, cyclopentasiloxane, glycerin, propylene glycol, dimethicone, cetyl peg/ppg-10/1 dimethicone, isododecane, mica, peg/ppg-18/18 dimethicone, disteardimonium hectorite, sodium chloride, sorbitan sesquioleate, tribehenin, safflower seed oil, phenoxyethanol, polysilicone-11, methicone, hdi/trimethylol hexyllactone crosspolymer, silica, dimethicone/ vinyl dimethicone crosspolymer, propylene carbonate, tocopheryl acetate, aloe leaf extract, tea leaf extract, mineral oil, disodium edta, fragrance, bht, matricaria flower extract, tea tree leaf oil [may contain: titanium dioxide (ci 77891), iron oxides (ci 77491, ci 77492, ci 77499)].

Here is a mix of silicones, mica, wax and pigments. This product is likely to be good at hiding scars.

Unfortunately, there are no great products to help erase scars or prevent them from forming in the first place. Surgeons are mostly interested in fixing the big problem and the creation of small scars are an accepted part of the procedure. Generally, surgeons will recommend silicone products like Mederma, while also letting you know that this type of product does *not* improve outcomes in new or old scars. SAS products should help prevent scar formation (Restoration Cream) and may help alleviate old scars (Scar Vanishing Gel) but the main factor is the genetics of your skin and how it will interact with the actives in these two products.

Our products will not *hide* scars because they haven't been formulated for this purpose. They're not thick creams and they don't contain pigments to mimic the natural color of the skin. What do they do, then? Let's look at the ingredient lists:

Restoration Cream: distilled water, jojoba seed oil, lactobacillus/ kelp ferment filtrate, sorbitol, butylene glycol, cetyl alcohol, glyceryl stearate, PEG-100 stearate, stearyl alcohol, sesame seed oil, sweet almond oil, avocado oil, pomegranate seed oil, rosehip seed oil, hydrolyzed collagen, *Laminaria Japonica* extract, gotu kola extract, carnosine (L-), ceramides, aloe vera polysaccharides, indian frankincense extract, coconut endosperm, hyaluronic acid, copper peptide (copper tripeptide-1, GHK), glycerol, epidermal growth factor (sh-Oligopeptide-1, EGF), tocotrienols, alpha-D-tocopherol, astaxanthin, lycopene, lutein, alpha lipoic acid, beta carotene, polysorbate 20, citric acid, dimethicone, carbomer, aminomethyl propanol, phenoxyethanol, methylparaben, propylparaben.

Restoration Cream's key ingredient is epidermal growth factor, a naturally occurring protein capable of stimulating cellular proliferation and differentiation. For more about EGF see Chapter 12.

SAS Restoration Cream will prevent water loss from the damaged skin, allowing the skin to repair itself. Within that repair zone, epidermal growth factor will be directing the show while other actives decrease inflammation and prevent the formation of an excess of free radicals.

SAS makes a Scar Vanishing Gel, which should help with scars of all kinds. Remember that your skin is no longer that of a baby, so your aim should not be to acquire the smooth surface of the photo-shopped celebrity but an overall better-looking adult skin. Scars can be the result of minor accidents and teenage acne, the kind of imperfections that we see better than anybody else. We may wish to start a new year feeling like new, but our skin looks much the same as last year, or older! Have a look at your old scars and spots and decide whether you want to do something about them.

SAS Scar Vanishing Gel: lactobacillus/kelp ferment filtrate, glycerin, oleuropein, tetrahydrocurcuminoids, aloe powder extract, green tea EGCG, apigenin, *Centella asiatica,* luteolin, epidermal growth factor (sh-oligopeptide-1, EGF).

Healing and scar remodeling are complicated processes, but this gel works to reduce scarring by improving hydration, switching the type of collagen made in the dermal matrix, and decreasing inflammation. Glycerin and aloe vera help by improving hydration of the skin, *Centella asiatica* extract helps by switching the type of collagen made in the dermal matrix, and apigenin decreases inflammation, but much remains to be studied. New scars should respond to SAS Scar Vanishing Gel after a few weeks, but older scars will respond more slowly. For older scars, you should feel a softening of the scar after a month or so and see changes in appearance occurring in the following months.

References:

Fujimura T. (2002) Treatment of human skin with an extract of *Fucus vesiculosus* changes its thickness and mechanical properties. J Cosmet Sci. 53:1-9.

O'Leary R, Rerek M, Wood, EJ. (2004) Fucoidan modulates the effect of transforming growth factor (TGF)-Beta1 on fibroblast proliferation and wound repopulation in in vitro models of dermal wound repair. Biol Pharm Bull.27:266-270.

Widgerow, AD; Chait, LA; Stals, PJ; Stals, R; Candy, G (2009) Multimodality scar management program. Aesth Plast Surg (2009) 533-543

Chapter 11: Skin non-problems

Myth: Skin should be smooth

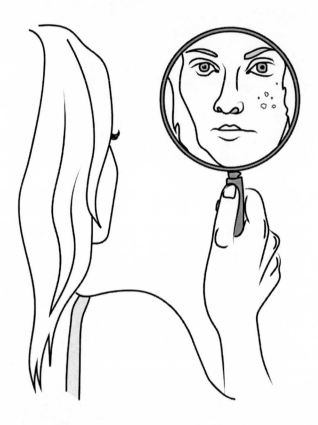

I keep coming back to this subject again and again. Why? Because about one half of the emails I receive have to do with pores: *blocked* pores, *large* pores, or *ugly* pores, etc. It seems that we are obsessed with pores! But this isn't surprising. Photography tricks, including sophisticated lighting and editing with Photoshop, have convinced consumers that they can have *baby smooth* skin. We can't. Look at any picture of a celebrity *au naturel* and compare it with a published photograph and you'll see the difference. A Google search of "celebrities without makeup" is enlightening.

What to do with pores? First, try doing nothing. If you don't have comedones, blackheads or acne lesions, your pores are NOT clogged and you should leave them alone. If you get the idea to look at your face in a magnifying mirror, the pores may look *full*. This may be an optical illusion, or maybe there is some leftover makeup or whatever. Just throw away the magnifying mirror and learn to enjoy your body as it is. Please don't squeeze pores, you may be lucky, but many people scar and get hyperpigmentation when they squeeze, depending on how their skin reacts to stress. Moreover, pore-squeezing could be considered an *entry-level* activity to dangerous OCD (obsessive compulsive disorder) that could later worsen and get into skin-picking. The *least* you can expect from pore squeezing is *increased* sebum secretion and pore *enlargement*.

False advertising makes us buy products that can't possibly have the effect advertised, which was obtained with photo editing and not with the product they are selling. But, most importantly, someone convinced that baby smooth skin is possible may try other, dangerous experimental treatments that could lead to permanent disfiguration.

Cellulite

Most of us know what cellulite looks like, but let me assure you that it is NOT a disease. Still, I managed to find a review on cellulite published in a relatively obscure medical journal (European Journal of Dermatology and Venereology, 2000, 14: 251-262). Despite the lack of recognition of cellulite in the medical field, this "condition" managed to gather a few medical-sounding names, like gynoid lipodystrophy, nodular liposclerosis, oedemato-fibrosclerotic panniculopathy and panniculosis. Skin care can make anything sound like a disease when they use Latin sounding names, but again, cellulite is not a disease. It has also been called "mattress skin" and "orange peel skin" to describe the superficial undulations of the skin.

Cellulite will happen to most women, so it is not an abnormal condition. As we age, our skin is no longer able to stretch smoothly over subcutaneous fat deposits, and that is NOT a disease. But just as we don't like wrinkles, we don't like cellulite. Is there anything that can be done? Cosmetic surgery can alleviate the problem by either injecting fat (yes!) in the "valleys" or doing liposuction in the "hills". Surgery may help, or not, but any positive effect is likely to be temporary.

There is something else that can be done without the risk and expense of cosmetic surgery. You can try to get that dormant, subcutaneous fat to enter back into your body metabolism. You can also increase the elasticity of your skin so that it will be able to cope with the increased fat volume. You could add some acetyl carnitine to our Vitamin A Cream. Caffeine will get rid of some water and wake up sleepy cells. It acts directly on fat cells by interacting with receptors and breaking down fats for local respiration or to be exported for use by the muscles.

Chapter 12: Good news: You *can* turn back the clock

Myth: There's a *magic bullet* in skin care

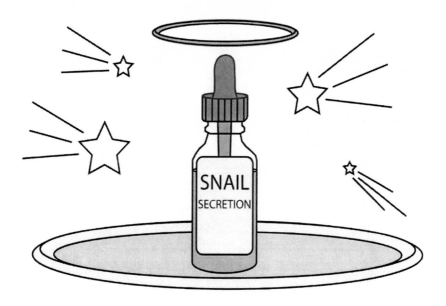

There is *no* magic bullet; no single ingredient is going to rejuvenate your skin ON ITS OWN. Your skin is a very complex system and has complex requirements. As you age, your body starts to *shortchange* the skin, even when you are eating a healthy diet and taking your multivitamins. Simply put, fewer blood vessels reach your dermis to deliver nutrients to the skin. Your skin is regularly starved of what it needs, so the addition of just one ingredient will not make a big change. Why? Because as soon as your skin has enough of ingredient A, the lack of another ingredient, B or C, will limit the capacity of your skin to regenerate.

What to do then? The solution is to give your skin plenty of nutrients, especially those your body cannot make, like essential fatty acids and essential amino acids. Any product that promises miracle results with one miracle ingredient is a lie.

Limiting factors in skin care

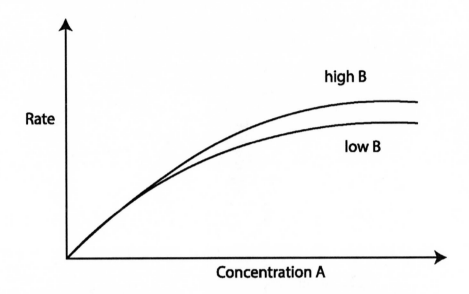

The graph above describes most biological processes that depend on the supply of nutrients or substrates. Let's use the graph to describe, for example, the division of skin cells, a process we want to promote in our aging skin.

Do the cells need glucose? OK, let's give them glucose and division rate should increase…. but only up to a point, because when the cells have enough glucose, the division rate will stop increasing. Maybe what they need at this point is an amino acid, say, proline? Let's add it. Division rate will increase but not "forever," not proportionally to the addition of proline because as soon as there is enough proline, another nutrient will become "limiting."

If you look at skin from this point of view, and we should because the skin is a biological system that responds in this manner to the addition of nutrients, then the "magic ingredient" approach of most skin care companies looks like nonsense (and it is nonsense). Even assuming that the kin of all the clients will be in need of the same nutrient, be it an amino acid, a sugar, a vitamin, whatever, it should be apparent that there is a certain amount of that ingredient that will benefit the skin and, after it is supplied, something else, not the ingredient advertised as magic, will be required.

This is why SAS products contain so many actives. For example our hair care serum contains keratinocyte growth factor (KGF) a powerful growth factor that will signal the keratinocytes in the scalp that they should multiply and produce hair. In addition, you also need to provide the keratinocytes with the building blocks they need so that that they can follow the instructions given by KGF. This is where amino acids, sugars, vitamins and more are required, and you will find a lot of them in the serum.

The complexity of biological processes is another reason why we focus each of our products on a particular issue, but are still attentive to the whole of the skin's biology. What's the point of killing acne bacteria with powerful oxidants when those oxidants will accelerate skin aging? Instead, we look at the whole picture and aim for long term results.

Aging skin: Can you turn back the clock?

The most visible manifestations of skin aging are wrinkles and sun spots. These are changes we can see with the naked eye but they are caused by microscopic changes in the structure of skin as well as subtle changes in the biochemical composition of the skin. *If* we could change these structural manifestations and return the skin to a physiology that resembles that of younger skin, we could argue that we would be *turning back the clock*. This is not just theory, as many clients of Skin Actives Scientific can attest to; it is a fact that many of these changes can indeed be reversed in such a way that the visual manifestations of aging are reversed to some extent. You can rejuvenate the skin by protecting it from further damage and by providing tools to reverse damage inflicted by age and the environment on cellular DNA. It is *crucial* that you protect your skin's stem cells, which will allow this most important human organ to heal and regenerate.

The temporary activation of the enzyme telomerase may extend the number of times a cell can divide before division stops, but this will be of no help to your skin if the stem cells in it are significantly damaged by ultraviolet (UV) radiation and other stressors. The objective of a *rejuvenating* cream should be to promote the skin's own healing powers by protecting its stem cells and supplying active ingredients known to help repair DNA mutations. Let's look at how skin anatomy is modified by aging.

Skin structure

We take our skin for granted, we don't think of our skin unless it gets cut or damaged in some way. But learning about the skin's structure and complexity can help us take care of it so that it can continue doing its job for many years.

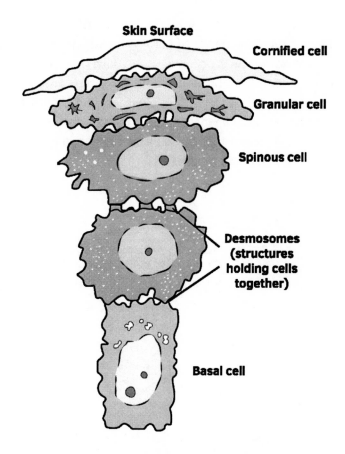

Skin Surface

Cornified cell

Granular cell

Spinous cell

Desmosomes (structures holding cells together)

Basal cell

How skin cells change shape and structure as they become the different layers of the skin. Cornified cells (corneocytes) are dead cells, but together they make a layer (horny layer, stratum corneum in Latin) that prevents water loss and the entry of microbes.

How cells change as they progress through the epidermis

The epidermis is divided into several layers where cells are formed through cell division (mitosis) at the inner layers. They move up the strata changing shape and composition as they differentiate and become filled with keratin. The cells eventually reach the top layer called the *stratum corneum* and are desquamated, or sloughed off. This process is called *keratinization* and takes place within weeks;

the outermost layer of the epidermis consists of 25 to 30 layers of dead cells. A structural matrix of keratin makes this outermost layer of the skin almost waterproof, and along with collagen and elastin, gives skin its strength. Ceramide is another main component of the *stratum corneum*. Together with cholesterol and saturated fatty acids, ceramide creates a water-impermeable, protective coating to prevent excessive water loss due to evaporation, as well as a barrier against the entry of microorganisms.

How the skin ages

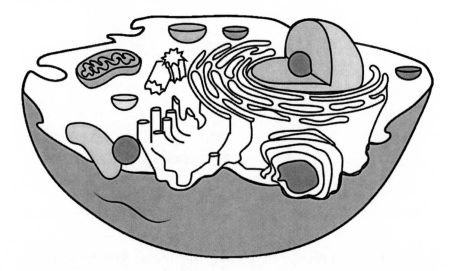

In the cell, the many subcellular compartments interact with each other and the complex membrane systems make these interactions possible. Aging affects all of the cell compartments and the membranes in many ways.

The visible differences between the skin of a young person and the skin of an elderly person are the superficial expression of major changes in the anatomy, physiology and biochemistry of the skin that occur as we age. As skin ages, one may expect: wrinkles, sun spots, decreased elasticity, decreased efficacy of the skin as a barrier, decreased ability to protect from UV rays, decreased ability to protect from temperature changes, diminished immune response, slower healing, and decreased ceramides and cholesterol content in the *stratum corneum.*

Some changes that we may attribute to skin aging are in fact related to the loss of fat under the skin. This distinction is important, because fat tissue is not easily manipulated by targeting skin metabolism.

A marked increase in the susceptibility to skin infections and malignancies has been observed in older humans, indicating that skin immunity becomes defective with age. Loss of effectiveness of the skin barrier probably has many causes, but one of them may be the decrease in ceramides that comes with aging.

Knowing that ceramides play a major role in the outer layers of the skin, providing resistance to water loss, it becomes apparent that there are two ways to address this problem: one is to provide the inner skin layers with fatty acids, the substrate they use to make ceramides. The other is to apply on the skin's surface extra ceramides or other waxy-like substances to prevent water loss.

What happens in our skin when we get a sun spot (solar lentigo)?

And what has changed in the cells involved? Ultraviolet (UV) radiation has caused so many changes, at so many levels, that I will only mention a few of them. Sun spots, or solar lentigos, are induced by mutations caused by past exposure to UV, leading to the characteristic increase in melanin production. Hyperpigmentation (increased melanin accumulation) is accompanied by decreased proliferation and differentiation of keratinocytes, and chronic inflammation. In a solar lentigo, the expression of genes related to inflammation, fatty-acid metabolism and melanocytes increases, and expression of filaggrin and involucrin decreases; cornification (the final stage of keratinization when cells become tough protective layers) is decreased. One crucial mutation is that of the fibroblast growth factor receptor 3 protein, which spans the cell membrane, so that one end of the protein remains inside the cell and the other end projects from the outer surface of the cell. This positioning of the protein allows it to interact with specific growth factors outside the cell and to receive signals that control growth and development. Solar lentigos are also different in their anatomy, the undulations of the dermoepidermaljunction (rete ridges) are elongated and there is an accumulation of abnormal elastin (actinic elastosis).

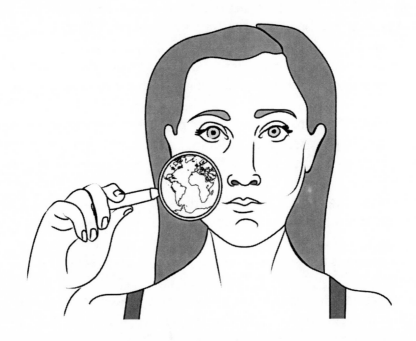

Sun damaged skin looks like a map, with dark islands, small areas of homogeneous pigmentation and spots that seem not white but almost lack the nice color of melanin, a situation that becomes more evident after exposure to the sun that, decades ago led to a smooth beautiful tan. The hands, subject to more stress of all kinds than any other part of the body, are not only more wrinkled but more irregular in their pigmentation. The loss of pigmentation is probably related to DNA mutations, just like the hyperpigmentation. But we can also look at a somewhat similar situation in the scalp, where loss of antioxidant enzymes results in loss of pigmentation in the hair.

What makes a wrinkle?

The epidermis becomes thinner during aging; this thinning is stronger in the deepest portion of the wrinkle, sometimes accompanied by a reduction of the number of cellular layers. The dermis-epidermis junction, i.e. the area of tissue that joins the epidermal and dermal layers of the skin, becomes flatter. The dermis and hypodermis become atrophied during aging, with a decrease in collagen, certain glycosaminoglycans and the adipose tissue of the hypodermis. Conversely, there is an increase in elastin, often with a distorted structure and impaired function.
The changes in cell morphology and biochemistry are accompanied by major structural and functional changes that occur in the dermal *extracellular matrix* where fibrillar collagens, elastic fibers and proteoglycans provide tensile strength, resilience (recoil) and hydration, respectively.

Skin proteins get glycosylated (sugar molecules are attached to the amino acids), modifying structure and function; in people with diabetes. The presence of higher glucose concentrations in blood accelerates this process and the damage it causes.

The activity of matrix metalloproteinases (MMPs) that break down skin proteins increases as a response to UV radiation.

The number of blood vessels reaching the skin (vascularization) decreases, and this brings a decrease in the supply of nutrients to the skin. This is why our products contain so many nutrients, including vitamins, amino acids, hyaluronic acids, etc., in order to compensate as much as possible for this loss.

Independently of the damage caused by UV radiation, some changes are intrinsic to aging and happen all over the body, not just in the skin. Cells age, mutations accumulate, mitochondria age, cells divide more slowly, metabolism slows down and the turnover of macromolecules slows down.

Trying to rejuvenate your skin? What will *NOT* work

Miracle ingredients (the ONE that will make you young again!) work only for marketing. There isn't a single chemical that can reverse aging all by itself. Why? Because aging affects many processes and structures, not just a single one.

One ingredient proclaimed by its advocates (and salespeople) as a "miracle ingredient" is copper peptide. In this case, copper tripeptide may help healing. Unfortunately, marketers have helped spread misinformation about this ingredient which is often used at concentrations that will *accelerate skin aging* rather than help.

Fast and furious solutions sold by the industry include devices that use light to heat skin cells when absorbed by water. Heating leads to inflammation, which plumps the skin temporarily, while causing long-term damage. Laser energy can be useful at killing damaged (pre-cancerous) cells but will not, in itself, rejuvenate the skin.

Cosmetic surgery

For skin rejuvenation, don't look at cosmetic surgery. Cosmetic surgery does not change older skin, indeed, cutting "extra" skin and tightening the rest does not restore a younger look but leads instead to a face that looks unnatural, almost like a mask. Moreover, if for some good reasons you decide to go the plastic surgery route, you still need to improve skin physiology, because older skin does not heal well or fast.

Dermal fillers

Dermal fillers are injectable chemicals that provide bulk under the skin to "fill" wrinkles and other depressions. The most common products are derivatives of hyaluronic acid modified chemically to delay breakdown by skin enzymes. The effectiveness of this method depends on the skills of the practitioner and the reaction (sometimes bad) of the individual's body to the material injected.

Botulinum toxin

Botulinum toxin is a neurotoxic protein produced by the bacterium *Clostridium botulinum*. The toxin treats wrinkles by immobilizing the muscles which cause wrinkles. It is not suitable for the treatment of *all* wrinkles, just for the glabellar lines (between the eyebrows) in adults. It is imperative that anyone considering "getting botox" read about the side effects and signs of an allergic reaction so the risks are fully comprehended.

Turning back the clock the SAS way

Skin Actives Scientific makes skin care products that are special because we use science to solve problems. It is true that these days we find scientific jargon used in practically all advertising for skin care, but when you read the ingredient list you will find out that, actually, the science is only being used for advertising. This is a terrible loss because there is a lot that is known about the skin and how it can be improved.

At Skin Actives we review scientific and industry literature to find the best skin care ingredients. We are not distracted by myths, fancy stories or scientific-sounding jargon; we evaluate information using scientific reasoning. In addition, we use advanced biochemical methodology to produce proteins that are beneficial to the skin or even prepare subcellular fractions if they are needed. We have the expertise to decide what ingredients can benefit the skin, find the best quality ingredients available, and if they are not available to purchase, we can synthesize them.

The following are *some* of the actives that can help restore cell function. For a more complete list, please see our glossary. It would not be useful to list all the ingredients that can help with skin aging and sun damage, so I chose a few whose mechanisms of action are better known.

Epidermal Growth Factor: the closest you can get to a miracle ingredient

A good example of an active that has been discussed in articles published in peer-reviewed scientific journals is epidermal growth factor (EGF). There are more than 50,000 pieces of scientific literature that document the activity of EGF. What is a growth factor? Growth factors are naturally occurring proteins capable of stimulating cellular proliferation and cellular differentiation. Growth factors bind to specific receptors on cell surfaces and are important for the regulation of a variety of cellular processes. Among the practical uses of EGF are its use in accelerating healing of the skin and cornea (the outside coating of the eyeball). EGF was the first growth factor to be discovered and studied, but many more factors have been found since then.

In 1986, Stanley Cohen received the Nobel Prize for his work elucidating the role of EGF in the regulation of cell growth and development. This small protein (only 53 amino acids) was found to enhance epidermal growth and keratinization. Work by Cohen and his collaborators demonstrated that EGF directly stimulated the proliferation of epidermal cells, and this stimulatory action of EGF did not depend on other systemic or hormonal influences. Cells that respond to EGF do so because they have receptors on the cell membrane that recognize the factor which has been produced by cells that may be near or far from the target cell. The binding of the growth factor to the receptor initiates a cascade of molecular events that will eventually lead, among other effects, to cell division. Among the practical uses of EGF are its use in accelerating healing of skin and corneas. Although EGF was the first growth factor to be discovered and studied, many more factors have been found since then. These growth factors differ in size and structure, and as a consequence, in the receptors and types of cells that recognize them, and the effects they have on the target cell. Not all growth factors are suitable for skin care; some of them can have unwanted effects on normal skin.

Menopause and hormones

Women who have decided not to go for hormone replacement therapy (HRT) after menopause may expect slow changes in their bodies, including, for example, loss of bone density, but many are taken by surprise by the negative changes they see in their skin and hair. What happened? Our skin has receptors for estrogen, and when the estrogen levels decrease with menopause, skin and hair age very quickly because estrogen is not there anymore to pass on messages to the skin and scalp cells.

Skin collagen content, skin thickness and forearm bone mineral content in postmenopausal women show similar declines of between 1-2% per year after menopause. We can't consider these declines in connective tissue structure and function abnormal, because all women who live to a certain age will eventually experience them. But *normal* does not mean *acceptable*. Now that age expectancy has increased by *decades*, women have the right to be annoyed at this inconvenience that ages us too soon when we are living full and demanding lives. What was good for the cavewoman, who would be eaten by a lion before she turned 50, is not good enough for modern women. At least - not for me.

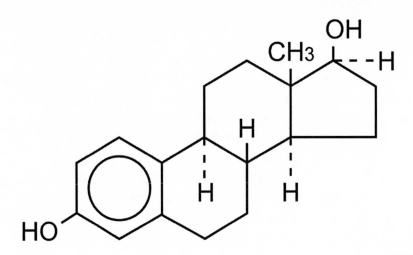

Estradiol: one of the female hormones that decreases drastically during menopause.

If you are not going to do HRT and you are not ready to see your skin and hair age practically overnight, there are some options. For example, you can go for skin and hair care products that will slow down, and even reverse, aging of skin and hair. Soy isoflavones will help a lot, as will nutrients such as: collagen peptides, hyaluronic acid, and various vitamins.

For hair, try our Hair Care Serum, it will stop hair loss and give you back some volume; look for apigenin in the ingredient list. We also offer a serum to recover eye lashes and eye brows. Be careful with the shampoo you use: you don't need the bubbles, and if the bubbles are there because of sodium lauryl sulfate, the price you will pay will be further hair loss. When it comes to your hair conditioner, look for nutrition for your scalp. We use Sea Kelp Coral for that and for softness as well.

For lips, see our Lip Care Kit, full of nutrients that nature *denies* to the lips of women over fifty. You can also try our Anti-Aging Cream, it contains a bit of everything and it works. This very complex cream contains soy isoflavones and resveratrol, which, among all of their properties, include the increase of phytoestrogenic activity.

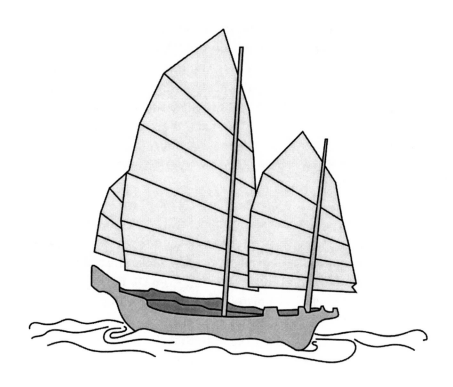

Xu Fu expedition for the elixir of life. Xu Fu was court sorcerer in China Qin Dynasty. He was sent to the eastern seas twice to look for the elixir of life; he did not find it.

Our Anti-Aging Cream contains soy isoflavones and resveratrol, but if you are over fifty you may need even more help. The new Elixir10 Phytoestrogen Booster is a mix of botanical extracts that can supply your skin and scalp with beneficial chemicals that will bind to the estrogen receptors left vacant by menopause.

Phytoestrogens are plant chemicals that can interact with two of the most important receptors of steroid hormones: the sex hormone-binding globulin and the cytosolic estrogen receptor. The chemical structure of phytoestrogens may vary greatly from estradiol, but a part of the molecule is similar enough to human estrogen to fool the receptor.

For those who think that maybe nature made these chemicals for our benefit, think again: they are part of the defense system against fungi. Also, in the 1940's, it was noticed that pastures of red clover, a phytoestrogen-rich plant, had effects on the reproductive ability of grazing sheep. It is likely that these plants evolved the biochemical pathways required to make these secondary metabolites to disrupt the hormonal balance in their predators, decreasing birth rates in sheep or whatever animal was having them for breakfast.

For SAS Elixir 10, we are using botanical extracts standardized for chemicals with estrogenic properties. As a bonus, many of these chemicals have other beneficial properties, including antioxidant and anticancer activities, and protection from UV damage. The ingredients are: soybean genistein, flax lignans, wild yam diosgenin, soybean daidzein, licorice extract, luteolin, resveratrol, apigenin, phloretin, kudzu puerarin. Please note that the beneficial properties listed below are *on top* of the estrogenic properties.

Kudzu puerarin. *Pueraria* is a rejuvenating folk remedy in Thailand, a tradition passed on from generation to generation. The Thai name is White Kwao Krua or Kwao Keur. Besides puerarin, the 8-C-glucoside of daidzein, kudzu contains other phytoestrogens, like miroestrol, deoxymiroestrol, daidzein, genistein, and coumestrol.

Genistein and daidzein stimulate the synthesis of hyaluronic acid. Genistein induces collagenation in soft tissue wound healing and inhibits tyrosine kinase. Daidzein activates all three peroxisome proliferator-activated receptors (PPAR) isoforms, a group of nuclear receptor proteins that function as transcription factors regulating the expression of genes, cellular differentiation, development, and metabolism.

Flax lignans are a class of phytoestrogens with antioxidant and cancer-preventing properties. Additionally, their skin strengthening properties will help prevent scarring and stretch marks.

Luteolin is a flavonoid with great properties: anti-aging, anti-itch, anti-inflammatory. It offers protection against lipid peroxidation and against protease activation caused by UV radiation.

Resveratrol (3,5,4'-trihydroxystilbene) is a polyphenolic antioxidant found in grapes and red wine. Resveratrol blocks UVB-mediated activation of the factor NFkappa-B, and this is the mechanism of protection against photocarcinogenesis. Besides direct antioxidant activity, plant polyphenols like resveratrol may benefit the skin with anti-inflammatory and wound-healing activity through their interaction with growth factor receptors and the cytoplasmic and nuclear pathways these receptors control.

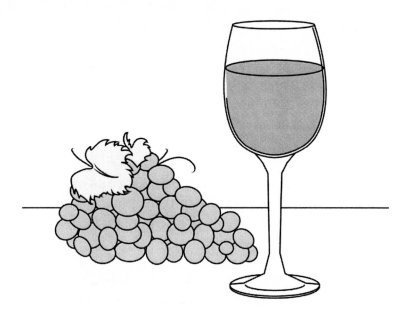

Apigenin is a phenolic flavonoid found in chamomile and many other plants. This antioxidant has anti-inflammatory, chemopreventive activity against skin cancer and prevents UVA and B induced skin cancer. It may also help prevent skin aging by UV through inhibition of metalloproteinases.

Apple Phloretin is an antioxidant and inhibits elastase activity. Phloretin has been shown to inhibit proliferation of breast cancer cells.

How vitamin A was found to be a vitamin

Vitamins are organic compounds that are essential to human metabolism, but that humans are unable to synthesize so they must be acquired through food. During evolution, we "simply" lost some enzymes required for their synthesis. Observations made before 1900 were that nutritional deprivation caused corneal ulcers, blindness, and high mortality and that an unknown substance present in milk and egg yolk was essential for nutrition. In the early 20th century it was found that this unknown substance was fat soluble. The growth-supporting "accessory factor" in milk and egg yolk became known as 'fat-soluble A' in 1918 and then 'vitamin A' in 1920. Further research, and huge advances in chemistry and biochemistry in the 20th century, elucidated the chemical structure of the molecule and eventually lead to its chemical synthesis in the laboratory.

One of the very important roles of vitamin A is to maintain epidermal integrity; it appears to maintain normal skin health by switching on genes and differentiating keratinocytes (immature skin cells) into mature epidermal cells.

After retinoic acid enters the cell, it binds to specific nuclear receptors. These "activated" nuclear receptors in turn bind to specific regulatory sequences (called retinoic acid response elements) in the DNA inside the nucleus and directly change gene expression of specific genes. Such changes in gene expression translate into changes in the production of proteins, and are responsible for the biological and therapeutic effects of retinoids.

In the 1970's, retinoic acid was used topically to control acne, and the effect was thought to be through reduction of sebum secretion.

In 1979 a synthetic derivative of vitamin A, 13-cis-retinoic acid (isotretinoin), was found to help with severe nodulocystic acne by reducing the size and secretion of the sebaceous glands. Although it is known that a certain fraction of isotretinoin breaks down to retinoic acid, the mechanism of action of the drug (original brand name Accutane) remains unknown and is a matter of some controversy. Isotretinoin also reduces bacteria in both the ducts and skin surface. This is thought to be a result of the reduction in sebum, a nutrient source for the bacteria.

The vitamin A found in animal sources, retinyl ester, is fat soluble. This is also the form of vitamin A we use in our Skin Actives products, and what is used in commercial vitamins. Retinol (the alcohol) and retinal (the aldehyde) are very unstable for commercial use and it makes sense to choose vitamins A more suitable than those as long as they have an equivalent activity.

Plants can be a source of pro-vitamin A because, if they contain alpha carotene, beta carotene, and other carotenes (as long as they contain the beta-ionone ring), the animals (including humans) that possess the enzymes required can transform these carotenoids into retinal.

Retinoids have significant effects on normal embryonic development. Retinoic acid has recently been characterized as a vertebrate morphogen, i.e. a signaling molecule that controls the spatial pattern of differentiation and the shape of the developing embryo. The potent teratogenic effects (malformations of the embryo) of retinoids are well established and are a consequence of their central role in morphogenesis. Isotretinoin is also a teratogen with a number of potential side-effects, so its use requires medical supervision and it is strictly controlled by law.

Retinol and its esters (retinyl acetate and retinyl palmitate) are converted into retinoic acid and bind to receptors on the nuclear membrane, and they exert their effects through these receptors.

Some effects of vitamin A deficiency are reversed by retinoic acid, but some organs (i.e. the retina and testes) require retinal or retinol, depending on the metabolism of the organ. Skin requires retinoic acid, not all of the effects of vitamin A require the same chemical form of vitamin A in every organ.

Hundreds of different chemicals share some of the activities of vitamin A, but their different structures also mean that side effects will be different. When it comes to synthetic derivatives, like isotretinoin, part of the effects may be due to its partial conversion in the body into retinoic acid but there is more to its mechanism of action which is still under investigation.

In general, retinoids tend to normalize cellular proliferation and differentiation. In human epidermis, low concentrations of retinoids generally increase keratinocyte proliferation, but high concentrations can be inhibitory. This effect is used in the treatment of psoriasis.

The benefits of topical tretinoin on human photodamaged skin were first observed in middle-aged women treated for persistent acne. These women described smoother, less wrinkled skin in addition to the clearing of acne. Improvements were noted in skin texture, wrinkling, pigmentation, and sallowness. Although these effects were first studied using tretinoin, retinyl acetate (vitamin A) has similar effects BUT without the irritation caused by tretinoin (and without the need for medical supervision required for the synthetic retinoid). Many people can't use topical tretinoin because of its side effects, which include skin irritation. We know that this is not a problem with retinyl esters, like retinyl acetate, because they work just as well or better, and because they don't have serious side effects and don't require medical supervision.

The lesson is that it is simply not worthwhile to suffer the side effects of tretinoin and other synthetic forms of vitamin A. SAS has ready-made products that deliver the benefits of retinyl acetate safely.

Reference:

J.J.J. Fu, G.G. Hillebrand, P. Raleigh, J. Li, M.J. Marmor, V. Bertucci,_P.E. Grimes, S.H. Mandy, M.I. Perez, S.H. Weinkle and J.R. Kaczvinsky (2010). A randomized, controlled comparative study of the wrinkle reduction benefits of a cosmetic niacinamide/ peptide/ retinyl propionate product regimen vs. a prescription 0.02% tretinoin product regimen. British J. Dermatology, 162: 647–654

Ascorbic acid

Ascorbic acid (and derivatives that our body can use) protects us from free radicals like those formed during exposure of our skin to UVA and UVB radiation. Ascorbic acid is also necessary to synthesize collagen, where it is required to hydroxylate the amino acid proline after synthesis of the protein. Scurvy is a syndrome of vitamin C deficiency and is related to defective collagen synthesis. Ascorbic acid is known to inhibit synthesis of melanin. This is probably because melanin is made by our skin in response to stress, and ascorbic acid is in the first line of defense, preventing the damage before melanin synthesis can be initiated. Ascorbic acid and its derivatives promote wound healing, control inflammation and reduce erythema (abnormal redness of the skin).

Hyaluronic acid

Glycosaminoglycans (GAGs) are produced by the body to maintain structural integrity in tissues and to maintain fluid balance. Hyaluronic acid is a type of GAG that promotes collagen synthesis, repair, and hydration. GAGs serve as a natural moisturizer and lubricant between epidermal cells. Because of its tremendous capacity to hold water, adding this active to your creams, lotions, gels or serums will help keep skin moist. Also, hyaluronidase in the skin will break this active down and the sugars released will be used to make new hyaluronic acid in our dermis, making this a truly great active ingredient!

Mitochondria Concentrate

SAS Mitochondria Concentrate obtained from cauliflower florets (rich in active mitochondria) supplies mitochondrial "spare parts" to the skin, not just a single component of the electron transport chain, like coenzyme Q10, but a myriad of lipids, cofactors and coenzymes that will be used by our skin's mitochondria.

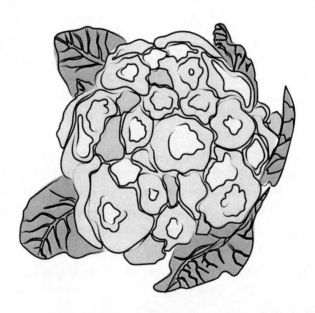

Cauliflower, it's good for you to eat, did you know it's great for topical skin care as well?

Glycan-7 Booster

Glycans can enhance immune response, which declines with age. Our Glycan-7 Booster is a combination of plant and fungal extracts that will promote and support the synthesis of collagen. This booster includes glycans from aloe, apple, larch, yeast, oat and brown algae which will help with the appearance of fine line and wrinkles.

The term glycan refers to a polysaccharide or oligosaccharide in which the subunits are linked via glycosidic bonds. In glycobiology, we are used to the idea that information is carried by our genes, and by the RNA and proteins resulting from the DNA-carried information. Information is also carried by glycans in processes like cell growth and apoptosis, folding and routing of glycoproteins, cell-cell interactions, and cell adhesion and migration.

Trichloracetic acid or TCA Spot Peel Kit (deep acid peel)

Because much of the damage done by UV radiation has to do with mutations, in theory we could eliminate the damage if we killed the mutated cells. The skin can heal itself using its own stem cells. The application of TCA onto skin to stimulate the stem cells can work if the cells killed are deep enough in the epidermis and the new *fresh* cells are recruited from areas where the stem cells have not been damaged. One problem with this approach is that it requires down-time or at least, time without being seen by anybody. Also, the treatment can be painful, because our skin is full of nerves whose job it is to let us know when our skin is hurt. Unless the area to be treated is very small (smaller than a quarter) this treatment should be administered by an experienced MD or a very experienced technician.

SAS ready-to-use products that can help keep your skin young and healthy:

Anti-Aging Cream

Our world class Anti-Aging Cream is geared towards women 50 and over, but is good for anybody over 35 who is worried about wrinkles and skin firmness. This cream is literally loaded with the best actives we could find to combat the effects of aging. These actives were hand-selected to work synergistically and address a wide variety of causes of aging, there is simply no product on the market that can compete with Skin Actives' Anti-Aging Cream.

This cream contains an active critical to mitochondrial activity, coenzyme Q10, Also, the mega-moisturizer hyaluronic acid, antioxidants galore (including glutathione and astaxanthin), and healing sea kelp bioferment. It contains resveratrol, which is a must for any anti-aging cream. Carnosine will prevent proteins like collagen from being glycosylated, decreasing elasticity of protein and skin. Alpha lipoic acid will act as an antioxidant and generate coenzymes essential for respiration. Receptors for estrogen (which decline slowly starting at about 35 or so), will be occupied by phytoestrogens from soy isoflavones, letting your skin know to slow down the aging process. Liquid crystal will provide cholesterol to your cell membranes and radiance that is more than just appearances. To round out the ingredient list, we included epidermal growth factor, an active you can only find in products priced at $150-600 per ounce. But even with EGF, you have to give the skin the building blocks it will need to build new proteins, lipids, cells, etc, and so here is what can help the rebuilding process:

Collagen Serum

One of our most complex ready-to-use products, our Collagen Serum promotes collagen synthesis in your skin. Use it to prevent skin aging, decrease wrinkles, increase elasticity, decrease acne scars, decrease stretch marks, and more!

ELS Serum

Use this to replenish lipids, the key to cellular function. ELS is one of our key products. It is essential for all skin types, especially those with dry skin, to soothe and moisturize. It will also help eliminate rough patches of skin affected by psoriasis. This serum contains the lipids all skin needs to maintain a healthy barrier against the environment. The objective of this *every lipid serum* (not literally *every* lipid, but close enough) is to provide an array of nutrients and antioxidants that your skin needs to stay healthy. Because this serum is formulated without water, it doesn't require preservatives - bacteria and mold can't live without water.

Revitalizing Night Cream

Use this cream to restore mitochondrial function. This cream remains the only skin care product anywhere to be formulated with plant mitochondria concentrate. Designed to slow the aging process by directly providing a full array of mitochondrial components to the skin, we can comfortably state that this cream is completely unique. For anyone 20 years of age and older, this cream will help slow skin aging by providing immune benefits, antioxidants and mitochondrial components to promote healthy skin.

UV Repair Cream

Here is a cream for anyone who wants to prevent and repair damage caused by the sun, in addition to providing many other benefits for their skin. This cream contains ingredients that are skin lightening, anti-aging, anti-inflammatory, anti-cancer, antioxidant, and much more!

Taking into account that most of the information on the subject of UV radiation's effects on skin was unavailable in the 50's and 60's - for many of us, our skin has already suffered the damage, and now we have to cope with the consequences. The objective of a *rejuvenating* cream should be to promote the skin's own healing powers by protecting its stem cells and supplying actives known to help repair DNA mutations This is why we created UV Repair Cream. This cream contains actives for everything, including anti-aging ingredients like resveratrol, lutein, astragalus, myricetin and silymarin. Skin lighteners like betulinic acid, niacinamide and tetrahydrocurcuminoids accompany others shown to help prevent cancer, like astragalus, betulinic acid, niacinamide, galangal, lycopene, sandalwood essential oil and more. This is a big bag of actives, which will work at every cellular level to restore youth and health to your skin. It is a great example of our approach: we throw at the skin every active for which there is scientific supporting evidence. As our clients find out when they try the products - the approach works.

Vitamin A Cream

Vitamin A is crucial for skin. This product is a great way to provide your skin with this beneficial active without irritation. When vitamin A is oxidized to retinoic acid, it is a growth factor for epithelial cells, where it binds to two different nuclear receptors to control gene transcription. Because of this, Vitamin A Cream is useful for a wide variety of skin issues. This cream can be used for acne, anti-aging, scarring and more. The regular use of Vitamin A Cream will help keep pores clear, improve wrinkles and keep skin renewed and feeling great.

If you have tried Retin-A and found that it was too irritating to your skin, this may be a good alternative. Research has shown that retinyl ester at 0.3% leads to significant improvement in wrinkles, comparable to those obtained by using the prescription medication retinoic acid (Retin-A).

Although some *building blocks* were added to enable the retinoid to do its job, we suggest you complement our Vitamin A Cream with Collagen Serum for even more skin benefits. If your skin is on the *dry* side, layer some Dream Cream on top of Vitamin A Cream for extra moisture.

Vitamin C Serum

Refresh your skin with our Vitamin C Serum. Although it might not be suitable for individuals with sensitive skin, the acidity of ascorbic acid will exfoliate and promote skin renewal. The vitamin C will help restore elasticity to aging skin, promote collagen synthesis, protect against UV damage, reduce redness, promote wound healing, and suppress melanin synthesis and more.

Prevention

The main agent of skin aging is UV radiation. Wear sunscreen, ours or any sunscreen that provides substantial protection. Remember that sunscreens do not prevent damage completely, but they extend the time of exposure before your skin gets damaged.
Avoid strong oxidants like benzoyl peroxide; they will age your skin. Look for alternatives that will control acne while protecting your skin from aging - try our Acne Control Kit.
Prevent damage by free radicals using our Antioxidant Day Cream and/or Antioxidant Serum and/or ROS*Terminator. You will need these products, especially if you live in a polluted city.
Protect your capillaries because they bring nutrients to your skin cells. Our Capillary Health Cream works to prevent and even reduce spider veins. Some of the actives in this cream have been used for centuries to help with varicose veins in different parts of the body, while others have been added more recently thanks to new scientific and clinical research.
Avoid inflammation as much as possible, and suppress inflammation without jeopardizing skin health with our Olive Anti-Inflammatory Cream. Do NOT use topical steroids long-term; they should only be used for emergencies, as they cause skin atrophy. Olive Anti-Inflammatory Cream includes the best anti-inflammatory actives available to help soothe the skin of individuals fighting psoriasis, eczema, atopic dermatitis, or other inflammatory conditions. Although the cause of each disorder may be different, the underlying inflammation common to all these afflictions should be alleviated using this product.

Summary

When it comes to the skin, because of its capacity for regeneration and self renewal, it *is* possible to turn back the clock. Avoid going the *quick-fix* route; you don't want to be a number in the statistics of plastic surgery or laser therapy gone wrong. I suggest you do it the Skin Actives Scientific way, preventing further damage and coaxing your skin into renewal with the help of the many active ingredients that science has discovered.

CPSIA information can be obtained
at www.ICGtesting.com
Printed in the USA
FSOW02n1324260117
29994FS